LEADING HEALTH INDICATORS 2030

Advancing Health, Equity, and Well-Being

Committee on Informing the Selection of
Leading Health Indicators for *Healthy People 2030*

Board on Population Health and Public Health Practice

Health and Medicine Division

A Consensus Study Report of

The National Academies of

SCIENCES · ENGINEERING · MEDICINE

THE NATIONAL ACADEMIES PRESS

Washington, DC

www.nap.edu

THE NATIONAL ACADEMIES PRESS 500 Fifth Street, NW Washington, DC 20001

This activity was supported by a contract between the National Academy of Sciences and the Department of Health and Human Services (HHSP233201400020B). Any opinions, findings, conclusions, or recommendations expressed in this publication do not necessarily reflect the views of any organization or agency that provided support for the project.

International Standard Book Number-13: 978-0-309-67187-3
International Standard Book Number-10: 0-309-67187-6
Digital Object Identifier: https://doi.org/10.17226/25682

Additional copies of this publication are available from the National Academies Press, 500 Fifth Street, NW, Keck 360, Washington, DC 20001; (800) 624-6242 or (202) 334-3313; http://www.nap.edu.

Printed in the United States of America

Suggested citation: National Academies of Sciences, Engineering, and Medicine. 2020. *Leading Health Indicators 2030: Advancing health, equity, and well-being*. Washington, DC: The National Academies Press. https://doi.org/10.17226/25682.

The National Academies of

SCIENCES • ENGINEERING • MEDICINE

The **National Academy of Sciences** was established in 1863 by an Act of Congress, signed by President Lincoln, as a private, nongovernmental institution to advise the nation on issues related to science and technology. Members are elected by their peers for outstanding contributions to research. Dr. Marcia McNutt is president.

The **National Academy of Engineering** was established in 1964 under the charter of the National Academy of Sciences to bring the practices of engineering to advising the nation. Members are elected by their peers for extraordinary contributions to engineering. Dr. John L. Anderson is president.

The **National Academy of Medicine** (formerly the Institute of Medicine) was established in 1970 under the charter of the National Academy of Sciences to advise the nation on medical and health issues. Members are elected by their peers for distinguished contributions to medicine and health. Dr. Victor J. Dzau is president.

The three Academies work together as the **National Academies of Sciences, Engineering, and Medicine** to provide independent, objective analysis and advice to the nation and conduct other activities to solve complex problems and inform public policy decisions. The National Academies also encourage education and research, recognize outstanding contributions to knowledge, and increase public understanding in matters of science, engineering, and medicine.

Learn more about the National Academies of Sciences, Engineering, and Medicine at **www.nationalacademies.org.**

The National Academies of
SCIENCES · ENGINEERING · MEDICINE

COMMITTEE ON INFORMING THE SELECTION OF LEADING HEALTH INDICATORS FOR *HEALTHY PEOPLE 2030*

GEORGE J. ISHAM (*Chair*), Senior Fellow, HealthPartners Institute
L. EBONY BOULWARE, Professor of Medicine; Chief, Division of General Internal Medicine; Vice Dean, Translational Science; Associate Vice Chancellor, Translational Research, School of Medicine, Duke University
GILBERT GEE, Professor, Department of Community Health Sciences, Fielding School of Public Health, University of California, Los Angeles
MARTHE R. GOLD, Senior Scholar, The New York Academy of Medicine
SHERI JOHNSON, Director, Population Health Institute, Associate Professor, Department of Population Health Sciences, School of Medicine and Public Health, University of Wisconsin–Madison
PAULA LANTZ, Associate Dean for Academic Affairs, Professor of Public Policy, Gerald R. Ford School of Public Policy, University of Michigan
DARCY PHELAN-EMRICK, Chief Epidemiologist, Baltimore City Health Department; Associate Scientist, Bloomberg School of Public Health, Johns Hopkins University
JONATHAN S. SKINNER, James O. Freedman Presidential Professor in Economics, Department of Economics, Dartmouth Institute for Health Policy and Clinical Practice, Geisel School of Medicine, Dartmouth College

Study Staff

ALINA B. BACIU, Study Director
CARLA S. ALVARADO, Program Officer
ANNA W. MARTIN, Administrative Assistant
ROSE MARIE MARTINEZ, Senior Director, Board on Population Health and Public Health Practice

Reviewers

This Consensus Study Report was reviewed in draft form by individuals chosen for their diverse perspectives and technical expertise. The purpose of this independent review is to provide candid and critical comments that will assist the National Academies of Sciences, Engineering, and Medicine in making each published report as sound as possible and to ensure that it meets the institutional standards for quality, objectivity, evidence, and responsiveness to the study charge. The review comments and draft manuscript remain confidential to protect the integrity of the deliberative process.

We thank the following individuals for their review of this report:

JOHN AUERBACH, Trust for America's Health
ANA DIEZ ROUX, Drexel University
CYNTHIA HAQ, University of California, Irvine
JEWEL MULLEN, University of Texas at Austin Dell Medical School
JOSÉ A. PAGAN, New York University
STEVEN M. TEUTSCH, University of California, Los Angeles, and University of Southern California

Although the reviewers listed above provided many constructive comments and suggestions, they were not asked to endorse the conclusions or recommendations of this report nor did they see the final draft before its release. The review of this report was overseen by **ERIC B. LARSON,** Kaiser Permanente Washington, and **JAMES S. HOUSE,** University of Michigan. They were responsible for making certain that an independent examination of this report was carried out in accordance with the standards of the National Academies and that all review comments were carefully considered. Responsibility for the final content rests entirely with the authoring committee and the National Academies.

Acknowledgments

The committee wishes to thank and acknowledge the many individuals and organizations that contributed to the study process and development of this report.

The committee appreciates the opportunity to assist the Department of Health and Human Services by providing advice on a key aspect of its *Healthy People 2030* effort.

The committee is grateful to experts who informed its deliberations through presentations and discussions that took place at the committee's public meetings. Four individuals provided background and insights about the Secretary's Advisory Committee on National Health Promotion and Disease Prevention Objectives for 2030 (SAC)—they included Deputy Assistant Secretary for Health Donald Wright, director of the Office of Disease Prevention and Health Promotion (ODPHP) Carter Blakey, ODPHP staff member Tiffani Kigenyi, and SAC co-chairs Dushanka Kleinman and Nico Pronk. Other speakers included Anita Chandra, Tom Eckstein, Marjory Givens, Kristen Lewis, Bobby Milstein, Ali Mokdad, Amy O'Hara, Carley Riley, Soma Saha, Brian Smedley, Sarah Treuhaft, and Steven Woolf.[1]

The committee thanks the National Academies of Sciences, Engineering, and Medicine staff who contributed to the production of this report, including study staff Alina Baciu, Carla Alvarado, Anna Martin, and Rose Marie Martinez. The committee's work received additional support from Andrew Koltun, Georgetown University medical student and

[1] Steven Woolf's slides were presented by Brian Smedley at the May 28, 2019, meeting.

population health scholar, who completed his summer practicum in the Health and Medicine Division (HMD). This project received assistance from Misrak Dabi (Office of Financial Administration); Clyde Behney, Tina Seliber, Lauren Shern, and Taryn Young (HMD Executive Office); and HMD communications staff, including Jeanay Butler, Sadaf Faraz, and Andrew Grafton.

Finally, the National Academies staff offers thanks to the executive assistants of committee members who provided scheduling support: Nancy Langer and Harriet Ware.

Contents

Boxes, Figures, and Tables

BOXES

FIGURES

TABLES

Summary

Beginning in 1979 and in each subsequent decade, the Department of Health and Human Services (HHS) has overseen the Healthy People initiative to set national goals and objectives for health promotion and disease prevention. Like its predecessors, *Healthy People 2030* (HP2030) includes a conceptual framework, a large set of objectives organized by topics, and a smaller set of high-level priority measures called Leading Health Indicators (LHIs). The committee that authored this report was asked to contribute two components to inform the HHS process illustrated in Figure S-1.

The HHS Office of the Assistant Secretary for Health has charged the National Academies of Sciences, Engineering, and Medicine committee to assist in the development of the LHIs for HP2030. The committee will develop (1) recommendations regarding the criteria for selecting LHIs and (2) a slate of LHIs that will serve as options for the Healthy People Federal Interagency Workgroup to consider as they develop the final criteria and set of LHIs for HP2030. The committee may identify gaps and may recommend new objectives for LHI consideration that meet the core objective criteria.

The committee's first report, *Criteria for Selecting the Leading Health Indicators for* Healthy People 2030 (NASEM, 2019c), was released in August 2019 and responded to the first part of the charge. The present report responds to the second part of the charge—putting forward a slate

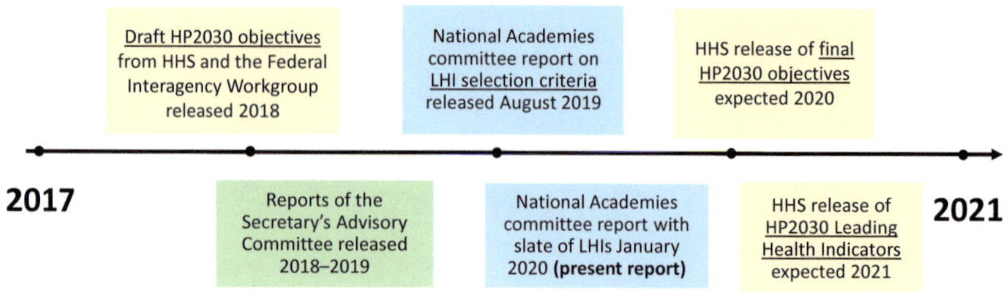

FIGURE S-1 Timeline and milestones in *Healthy People 2030*.
NOTES: National Academies reports are denoted in blue. HHS = Department of Health and Human Services; HP2030 = *Healthy People 2030*; LHI = leading health indicator.
SOURCE: NASEM, 2019c.

of LHIs based on its review of draft core objectives for HP2030[1] as well as identifying any gaps in the objectives and recommending additions.

The committee reviewed past and current Healthy People materials, both those developed by HHS and the current Secretary's Advisory Committee on National Health Promotion and Disease Prevention Objectives for 2030 (SAC), and prior National Academies reports.

FINDINGS AND RECOMMENDATIONS

In this report, **the committee recommends a set of 34 LHIs** organized by the 12 themes from the HP2030 Framework (see Table S-1).[2] The committee took three steps to assemble the most appropriate slate of LHIs:

1. It applied the criteria for LHI selection developed by the current SAC, along with the committee's own guidance about using alignment with the HP2030 Framework as a criterion.
2. In cases where a draft HP2030 objective was not available, it added a new objective if it met the SAC-described objective selection criteria.
3. It applied the SAC's criteria for the set of LHIs to the 34 LHIs collectively.

[1] According to HHS, the LHIs are to be selected from the HP2030 objectives, which had not been finalized at the time this report was prepared.

[2] The committee did not comment on targets for the LHIs or their associated objectives as that was not part of its charge.

The committee also made the following four findings regarding important topics that call for an LHI, but where the state of the field does not currently provide adequate support for such an indicator.

> Finding 1: The committee finds that a developmental objective of access to quality early childhood care and education could draw attention to the importance of starting early in placing children on the pathway to fourth grade reading proficiency and other measures of educational success.

> Finding 2: The committee finds that a developmental objective that tracks the cost of a "market basket" of widely used pharmaceuticals in comparison to their cost in other affluent nations could be informative to multiple stakeholders.

> Finding 3: The committee finds that a developmental objective on health care system administrative cost could provide a concrete proxy for health care spending more broadly, and could offer compelling information about health care cost that is easier to communicate to a range of audiences.

> Finding 4: The committee finds that the developmental objective per capita public health funding would elevate the profile of an often overlooked component of "health spending" writ large, and given the growing research and attention to data challenges, the measure's reliability and validity will likely be confirmed over the coming decade.

How the Proposed LHIs Differ from Past Sets

The Healthy People objectives and the Healthy People LHIs are used by agencies at all levels of government and in the private sector to guide various population health improvement agendas. The following examples illustrate the reach of the Healthy People effort in states and localities, such as Healthy Alaskans 2020, Healthy New Jersey, and Healthy Sonoma (California). HHS has been conducting a periodic series of webinars about the HP2020 LHIs, called "Who's Leading the Leading Health Indicators" featuring state, local, and private-sector (e.g., health system) initiatives and activities on specific LHIs.[3] The organization Grantmakers in Health

[3] See, for example, https://health.gov/news/events/2019/08/webinar-whos-leading-the-leading-health-indicators-nutrition-physical-activity-and-obesity-3 (accessed December 31, 2019).

developed a resource portfolio on the LHIs for HP2010.[4] The National Indian Health Board selected HP2020 LHIs that addressed the American Indian/Alaska Native population.[5]

The LHIs recommended in this report (see Table S-1) differ from past sets in several important ways. First, they are substantially reflective of the HP2030 Framework, which has health, equity, and well-being at its center. The LHI set recommended includes measures of well-being and health-related quality of life (these types of measures had been included in HP2020, but not among the draft core objectives for HP2030), and measures of equity that go beyond merely disaggregating data by race, ethnicity, sex, or geography and examine segregation and discrimination (see NASEM, 2017) for a discussion of poverty, racism, and discrimination as the root causes of health inequities.

Second, the LHIs include fewer health conditions; the need for parsimony and alignment with the HP2030 Framework required more measures of upstream factors that shape health (i.e., the causes of causes of poor health [Wilkinson and Marmot, 2003]). To keep the number close to 30 (the committee's original aim), members carefully considered the tradeoffs for each LHI selected. However, many important measures of health conditions (e.g., diabetes, chronic kidney disease, specific types of cancer) are included in the draft objectives for HP2030, and they will be monitored by different agencies at different levels of government in the course of HP2030 implementation even if they may not be included among the small number of final LHIs.[6]

Third, the recommended LHIs are to a lesser extent than ever before linked with the health care delivery system's capabilities and its metrics. Rather, many of the LHIs are indicators of how people live their lives in the United States—shaped by the broad context of policies, systems,

---

[4] See https://www.gih.org/publication/the-nations-leading-health-indicators-measuring-progress-taking-action (accessed December 18, 2019).

[5] See https://www.nihb.org/public_health/healthy_people_2020.php (accessed December 18, 2019).

[6] In winnowing the objectives to select LHIs the committee resolved to have certain indicators stand for a series of objectives that were of a similar nature. For example, hypertension was selected because for the prevalence to decrease many things need to happen: salt in the food supply and in people's diets needs to decrease; people need to have access to medical care, the medical care needs to be of good quality, people need to be able to afford the medications and/or change their behavior to achieve hypertension control (see, for example, CDC, 2011). Also, hypertension is a greater risk factor than cholesterol for cardiovascular disease (WHO, 2017). For many of the other clinical preventive services (colon, breast, and prostate cancers), although there is evidence of environmental risks (with tobacco being among the best understood), many of them and potential interventions are not as well elucidated or understood as for hypertension, perhaps making related measures less likely to meet the LHI criterion "actionable" (AACR, 2019).

TABLE S-1 Recommended Leading Health Indicators

No.	LHI Candidate	Measure (new objective, unless HP2030 draft core objective is listed, denoted by XX-2030-XX*)	HP2030 Framework Concepts (see Figure 1-1)
1	Life expectancy	Increase life expectancy (at birth)	Closing gaps: Health Equity
2	Child health	MICH-2030-02 Reduce the rate of all infant deaths	Health and Well-Being Across the Lifespan: Physical Health
3	Child health and well-being	Reduce the prevalence of one or more adverse childhood experiences (ACEs) from birth to age 17	Health and Well-Being Across the Lifespan: Mental Health
4	Self-rated health	Increase the mean healthy days (CDC HRQOL–14 Healthy Days)	Health and Well-Being Across the Lifespan: Physical Health
5	Well-being	Increase proportion thriving on Cantril's Self-Anchored Striving Scale	Health and Well-Being Across the Lifespan: Physical Health
6	Disability	Reduce the percentage of adults aged 65 years and over with limitations in daily activities	Health and Well-Being Across the Lifespan: Physical Health
7	Mental disability	Reduce the rate of mental disability	Health and Well-Being Across the Lifespan: Mental Health
8	Substance use	SU-2030-03 Reduce drug overdose deaths	Health and Well-Being Across the Lifespan: Physical Health
9	Unintentional injury deaths	IVP-2030-03 Reduce unintentional injury deaths	Increasing Knowledge and Action: Physical Health
10	All cancer deaths	C-2030-01 Reduce the overall cancer death rate	Health and Well-Being Across the Lifespan: Physical Health
11	Suicide	MHMD-2030-01 Reduce the suicide rate	Health and Well-Being Across the Lifespan: Mental Health
12	Firearm-related mortality	IVP-2030-12 Reduce firearm-related deaths	Health and Well-Being Across the Lifespan: Physical Health
13	Maternal mortality rate	MICH-2030-04 Reduce maternal deaths	Closing Gaps: Health Equity

continued

TABLE S-1 Continued

No.	LHI Candidate	Measure (new objective, unless HP2030 draft core objective is listed, denoted by XX-2030-XX*)	HP2030 Framework Concepts (see Figure 1-1)
14	Mental health	Reduce percentage of adults who reported their mental health was not good on 14 or more days in the past 30 days (i.e., frequent mental distress)	Health and Well-Being Across the Lifespan: Mental Health
15	Oral health access	OH-2030-08 Increase the proportion of children, adolescents, and adults who use the oral health care system	Health and Well-Being Across the Lifespan: Physical Health
16	Reproductive health care services	FP-2030-07 Increase the proportion of sexually active adolescents aged 15 to 19 years who use any method of contraception at first intercourse	Health and Well-Being Across the Lifespan: Access to Quality Public Health and Clinical Care Systems
17	HIV incidence	HIV-2030-03 Reduce the number of new HIV diagnoses among persons of all ages	Health and Well-Being Across the Lifespan: Physical Health
18	Tobacco	TU-2030-13 Reduce the use of any tobacco products by adolescents	Increasing knowledge and action: Evidence-based laws, policies, and practices
19	Obesity	NWS-2030-03 Reduce the proportion of children and adolescents aged 2 to 19 years who have obesity	Health and Well-Being Across the Lifespan: Physical Health
20	Alcohol use	SU-2030-13 Reduce the proportion of people with alcohol use disorder in the past year	Health and Well-Being Across the Lifespan: Physical Health
21	Immunization	Increase the proportion of 19–35-month-old children up to date on DTaP, MMR, polio, Hib, HepB; varicella, and pneumococcal conjugate vaccines	Increasing knowledge and action: Evidence-based laws, policies, and practices (also public health successes)
22	Hypertension rate	HDS-2030-04 Reduce the proportion of adults with hypertension	Health and Well-Being Across the Lifespan: Physical Health

TABLE S-1 Continued

No.	LHI Candidate	Measure (new objective, unless HP2030 draft core objective is listed, denoted by XX-2030-XX*)	HP2030 Framework Concepts (see Figure 1-1)
23	Ambulatory care-sensitive conditions/ avoidable hospitalization	Reduce discharges for ambulatory care-sensitive conditions per 1,000 Medicare enrollees (CMS-2)	Health and Well-Being Across the Lifespan: Access to Quality Public Health and Clinical Care Systems
24	Medical insurance coverage	AHS-2030-01 Increase the proportion of persons with medical insurance	Health and Well-Being Across the Lifespan: Access to Quality Public Health and Clinical Care Systems
25	Affordable housing	SDOH-2030-04 Reduce the proportion of all households that spend more than 30 percent of income on housing	Cultivating Healthier Environments: Social Environment
26	Environment	Improve the Environmental Quality Index	Cultivating Healthier Environments: Physical Environment
27	Environment	Lower the Heat Vulnerability Index	Cultivating Healthier Environments: Physical Health
28	Education	AH-2030-04 Improve the fourth grade reading level	Cultivating Healthier Environments: Social Environment
29	Poverty	SDOH-2030-03 Reduce the proportion of persons living in poverty	Cultivating Healthier Environments: Economic Environment
30	Food security	NWS-2030-01 Reduce household food insecurity	Cultivating Healthier Environments: Social Environment
31	Civic engagement	Increase the proportion of voting eligible population that votes	Cultivating Healthier Environments: Social Environment
32	Social environment	Lower the Neighborhood Disinvestment Index	Closing Gaps: Health Equity
33	Social environment	Reduce the level of residential segregation captured by the Index of Dissimilarity	Closing Gaps: Health Equity

continued

TABLE S-1 Continued

No.	LHI Candidate	Measure (new objective, unless HP2030 draft core objective is listed, denoted by XX-2030-XX*)	HP2030 Framework Concepts (see Figure 1-1)
34	Social environment	Reduce the level of residential segregation captured by the Isolation Index	Closing Gaps: Health Equity

NOTE: CHR = County Health Rankings; CMS-2 = a chronic conditions composite measure developed by Centers for Medicare & Medicaid Services; DTaP = diphtheria; Hep B = hepatitis B; Hib = Haemophilus influenzae type B; HIV = human immunodeficiency virus; MMR = measles, mumps, rubella.

* Items that include an acronym or abbreviation that represents the topic and the draft objective number, such as, "SU-2030-03: Reduce drug overdose deaths," are draft HP2030 objectives, which are listed in Appendix E. All others are new objectives.

social structures, and economic forces. This is true of many of the LHIs, including firearms-related mortality, deaths by suicide and drug overdose, maternal mortality, voting as a measure of civic engagement, and the health effects of climate change. Finally, the recommended LHIs are intended to balance those that operate and are measured at the individual level with those that operate and are measured at the environmental level (biological, physical, chemical, social).

1

Introduction

In 1979, Congress authorized the Secretary of Health and Human Services through Title XVII of the Public Health Service Act to set national disease prevention and health promotion goals and objectives. Starting with 1980 and for each subsequent decade, the Department of Health and Human Services (HHS) has launched and overseen a Healthy People initiative. Like its predecessors, *Healthy People 2030* (HP2030) includes a conceptual framework, a broad list of objectives organized by topics (objectives expected to be finalized by HHS in early 2020), and ultimately, a smaller set of high-level priority measures called Leading Health Indicators (LHIs) (see Figure S-1, reprised from NASEM, 2019c).

The National Academies of Sciences, Engineering, and Medicine convened a consensus study committee at the request of the Office of the Assistant Secretary for Health to provide advice on two components of the HP2030 effort. The Statement of Task is provided in Box 1-1. In May 2019, the charge was clarified slightly to add the following sentence: "The committee may identify gaps and may recommend new objectives for LHI consideration that meet the core objective criteria." This change was made in recognition that the Federal Interagency Workgroup (FIW), which would make final decisions about the LHIs, was instructed by HHS to draw the LHIs only from the core objectives for HP2030. A report from the Secretary's Advisory Committee on National Health Promotion and Disease Prevention Objectives for 2030 (SAC) had highlighted potential areas for adding to the draft core objectives to ensure the availability of appropriate candidates for LHIs (SAC, 2019). Given the revised charge to the committee and as the final core objectives will not be announced until

BOX 1-1
Statement of Task

The Department of Health and Human Services Office of the Assistant Secretary of Health requests that the National Academies of Sciences, Engineering, and Medicine convene an ad hoc committee to assist in the development of Leading Health Indicators (LHIs) for *Healthy People 2030*. The committee will develop (1) recommendations regarding the criteria for selecting LHIs and (2) a slate of LHIs that will serve as options for the Healthy People Federal Interagency Workgroup to consider as they develop the final criteria and set of LHIs for *Healthy People 2030*. The committee may identify gaps and may recommend new objectives for LHI consideration that meet the core objective criteria.

after this report is released, this report has drawn on the core objectives submitted for public review by HHS (2018), considered the recommendations of the SAC in its reports, and explained the committee's judgment in identifying new objectives that could serve as LHIs that best reflect the final HP2030 mission, vision, and framework (HHS, 2018).

THE COMMITTEE'S APPROACH

After starting its work in January 2019, the committee held three information-gathering meetings between February and May 2019—two were web-based and consisted of presentations from HHS and the leadership of the SAC and its relevant subcommittees, and one meeting took place at the Keck Center of the National Academies in Washington, DC, and included speakers from HHS and the SAC, as well as national experts on health metrics and data sources.[1] In addition to these, the committee held 19 virtual meetings to deliberate about report findings and recommendations.

The committee recognizes that the HP2030 is an enormous undertaking by HHS, the FIW, and the SAC. The effort has included multiple meetings of and reports from the SAC, an extensive and in-depth process by the FIW to substantially reduce the large number of objectives (1,200 for HP2020) to a more manageable set (355 draft core objectives, along with additional developmental and research objectives), and HHS's oversight of a complex, multi-component process that included gathering stakeholder input. The committee also appreciated the SAC's detailed

[1] See http://nationalacademies.org/hmd/Activities/PublicHealth/LeadingHealthIndicatorsForHealthyPeople2030.aspx (accessed January 2, 2020).

presentations and responsiveness in extensive conversations that occurred at the public meetings described above.

The committee approached the task by gathering information from several sources as inputs into its deliberations about an appropriately constructed, parsimonious, and balanced set of LHIs. Although it did not have the time or resources for a systematic search of the literature, the committee's information gathering involved a wide-ranging literature search. Sources included the reports and summaries of meetings of the SAC; presentations and materials from three information-gathering meetings; past Healthy People reports; articles from peer reviewed journals; reports, briefs, and white papers; and past reports from National Academies consensus committees.

As has been well documented in previous Institute of Medicine publications, health and related metrics have been proliferating for many years (IOM, 2011, 2015b), and the corresponding literature is vast. The committee focused primarily on highly reputable sources of metrics sets currently available to the field, some of which were presented by experts at its May 28, 2019, information-gathering meeting. Members also developed an efficient framework for reviewing and weighing that evidence, and on that basis, for coming to consensus around a set of indicators to put forward. This is discussed in Chapter 2.

On its review of the notes and slides from the June 2019 meeting of the SAC, the committee found the graphic designed to illustrate the HP2030 Framework (see Figure 1-1) to be a helpful tool that articulates and further explains the core focus of the HP2030 effort. Before viewing the SAC graphic, the committee had begun collecting other graphic representations of the multiple factors that contribute to health and well-being. These range from the World Health Organization (WHO) conceptual framework on the social determinants of health to the HP2020 social determinants of health graphic. The committee believes that other models, including those that are dynamic in the sense that they illustrate the relationship and effect of various factors to key outcomes of health and well-being, could be helpful toward operationalizing the themes and sub-themes[2] of the HP2030 graphic (see Figure 1-1). As an example, the WHO conceptual framework for action on the social determinants of health is intended to "highlight the difference between levels of causation, distinguishing between the mechanisms by which social hierarchies are created, and the conditions of daily life which then result" (WHO, 2010). The WHO framework can shed light on relationships among components of the HP2030 graphic, which appears to be primarily a graphic representation of the HP2030 narrative framework's list of foundational principles.

[2] The SAC and HHS call these "top-level concepts" and "sub-level concepts."

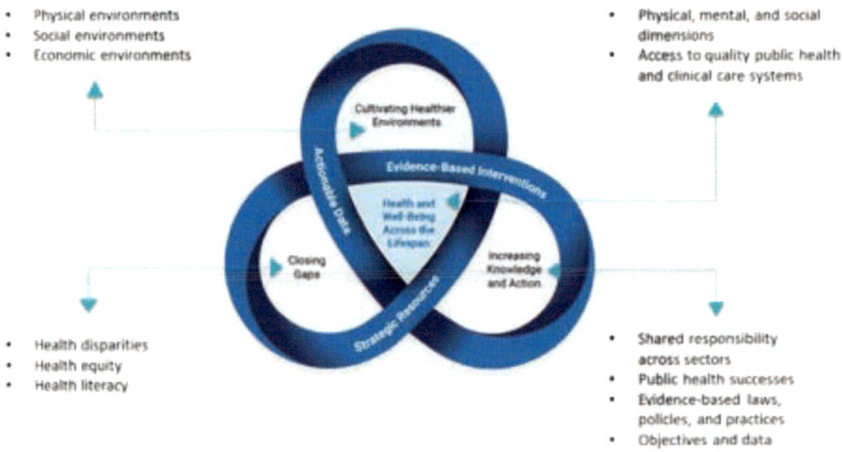

FIGURE 1-1 The *Healthy People 2030* Framework graphic.
SOURCES: SAC June 2019 meeting slides; ODPHP, 2019.

Another graphic, the National Institute on Minority Health and Health Disparities (NIMHD) Minority Health and Health Disparities Research Framework, offers an ecological model-informed framing of what it calls "levels of influence" along the top of the table—individual, interpersonal, community, and societal—and the "domains of influence" in the left-hand column—from the biological to the built environment.[3]

The set of LHIs proposed in this report is different from the HP2010 and HP2020 sets in several ways: it is reflective of the HP2030 Framework, it contains fewer measures of specific health conditions, and it is less closely linked with health care delivery system metrics and capabilities. To identify a set of indicators to serve as a North Star for national efforts to improve equitable health and well-being, in keeping with the priorities of the HP2030 Framework the composition of the LHIs measures needed to be rethought.

[3] Both WHO and NIMHD graphics are provided in Appendix C.

2

The Process for Identifying Candidate Leading Health Indicators

At its April 19, 2019, public information-gathering virtual meeting with the Secretary's Advisory Committee on National Health Promotion and Disease Prevention Objectives for 2030 (SAC) co-chairs and the co-chairs of the objectives and data subcommittees, the National Academies committee learned that the SAC intended for the Leading Health Indicator (LHI) selection criteria to be applied to all of the *Healthy People 2030* (HP2030) core objectives. The SAC developed two sets of criteria to be applied sequentially. In Phase 1, four criteria would be applied to rank the objectives (see Table 2-1). In Phase 2, the subset ranked highly in Phase 1 would undergo an iterative process of being assessed against four additional criteria for the set of LHIs. The iterative process would involve multiple considerations related to the Phase 2 criteria, which would mean that decision makers could add or remove some objectives from LHI consideration based on discussions about those considerations. In its report on the criteria for LHI selection, the National Academies committee recommended using the HP2030 Framework itself as Phase 0 in LHI selection (see Table 2-1).

The committee did not undertake a process that ranked each of the 355 draft core objectives for HP2030 on the LHI criteria. That is because the HP2030 objectives had not been finalized at the time the committee began its work and were not expected to be completed until much later. Thus, instead of obtaining a list of LHI candidates based on evaluating and rating each of the 355 draft core objectives, the committee used two approaches that integrated all LHI selection criteria (see Table 2-1) and the core objective selection criteria (see Box 2-1).

TABLE 2-1 Criteria for LHI Selection (Phase 0) Recommended in NASEM, 2019c; Phases 1 and 2 Developed by the SAC/HHS

Phase 0 (recommended in NASEM, 2019c; themes and subthemes drawn from the HP2030 Framework developed by the Secretary's Advisory Committee)	Phase 1 (developed by the Secretary's Advisory Committee)	Phase 2 (developed by the Secretary's Advisory Committee; edited for brevity below)
Alignment with the HP2030 Framework: Themes and Subthemes (the description in Figure 1-1) Closing Gaps • Health disparities • Health equity • Health literacy Cultivating Healthier Environments • Physical environments • Social environments • Economic environments Increasing Knowledge and Action • Shared responsibility across sectors • Public health successes • Evidence-based laws, policies, and practices • Objectives and data Health and Well-Being Across the Lifespan • Physical, mental, and social dimensions • Access to quality public health and clinical care	Apply the following criteria to the individual LHI candidates: • Public health burden—relative significance to the health and well-being of the nation • Magnitude of the health disparity and the degree to which health equity would be achieved if the target were met • The degree to which the objective is a sentinel or bellwether • Actionability	Apply the following criteria to the set of LHIs: • Balanced portfolio (health, well-being, across the lifespan) • Balance: common upstream root causes and high-priority health states • Amenable to interventions of different types (policy, environmental, systems) at all levels (e.g., national, state, local, and for the purpose of, including informing international comparisons) • Understandable, resonate with diverse stakeholders

BOX 2-1
Criteria for the *Healthy People 2030* Objectives (developed by the Secretary's Advisory Committee)

1. **Measurable.** The Core objective must be measurable by the data cutoff for inclusion in HP2030, which [is] mid-2019.

2. **Current Baseline Data.** The Core objective must reasonably be expected to have a baseline using data no older than 2015, and at least two additional data points during the HP2030 decade.

3. **National Importance.** The objective must be of national importance. To meet the "national importance" criterion, objectives should have a direct impact or influence on health, broad and comprehensive applicability, a substantial burden, and they should address a national health priority
   a. Direct impact or influence on health: Does this objective address an outcome or preventive/risk factor that has a direct impact on population health?
   b. Broad and comprehensive applicability: Does this objective address a broad health concern or topic that is applicable to a large part of the population, as opposed to being limited to more narrowly defined groups?
   c. Substantial burden: Does this objective address a health concern that represents a substantial impact or potential impact on the health or well-being of an individual or on a population?
   d. National (not just federal) public health priority: Does this objective address a public health priority of the Department of Health and Human Services, national prevention initiatives, other national indicator projects, and efforts at the state, local, and tribal level across the country?

4. **Evidence Base.** The objective should have a known evidence base and identified evidence-based interventions to improve outcomes. The effectiveness of the objectives was rated based on the scale used in *Healthy People 2020* to rate evidence-based resources[a] on the website.

5. **Health Equity and Disparities.** The objectives should address health disparities and/or support achieving health equity. Health equity and disparities have been an important part of the Healthy People initiative since *Healthy People 2000*. Health equity is defined by the HHS Office of Minority Health (OMH) as, "Attainment of the highest level of health for all people. Achieving health equity requires valuing everyone equally with focused and ongoing societal efforts to address avoidable inequalities, historical and contemporary injustices, and the elimination of health and healthcare disparities." OMH defines health disparities as, "A particular type of health difference that is closely linked with social or economic disadvantage. Health disparities adversely affect groups of people who have systematically experienced greater social and/or economic obstacles to health and/or a clean environment based on their racial or ethnic group; religion; socioeconomic status; gender; age; mental health; cognitive,

continued

BOX 2-1 Continued

sensory, or physical disability; sexual orientation; geographic location; or other characteristics historically linked to discrimination or exclusion." Objectives are also considered for inclusion, based on the expectation that the data source is able to track the following population-level data.

- Sex
- Race/Ethnicity
- Age
- Educational Attainment
- Family Income
- Health Insurance Status
- Geographic Location or Region
- Marital Status
- Sexual Orientation
- Gender Identity
- Disability Status

[a] See https://www.healthypeople.gov/2020/tools-resources/Evidence-Based-Resources#ratings (accessed May 29, 2019).
SOURCE: SAC, 2018a.

This chapter provides an overview of the process undertaken by the committee to review and weigh the available evidence to inform the selection of a set of candidate LHIs. The committee's present work builds on the first report on criteria for LHI selection (see Box 2-2 for the report's findings and recommendations).[1]

This report proposes LHIs—and where appropriate, new topics and objectives related to LHIs for which there were no extant draft core objectives—that reflect the intent of all components of the HP2030 Framework and criteria for core objective selection. It identifies areas where measures appropriate to serve as LHIs are available for making international comparisons. Lastly, it applies the LHI selection criteria described earlier.

The committee reviewed a large group of well-validated measure sets as described next. It then (1) drew on those existing sources to identify priority candidates for LHIs (i.e., the top-down procedure; see Chapter 3) and (2) applied a systematic approach to selecting from among the current draft core objectives by comparing them to the results of (1) (i.e., the bottom-up procedure, described in Chapter 4).

[1] The entire report is available for free download at https://www.nap.edu/25531 (accessed August 20, 2019).

BOX 2-2
Findings and Recommendations from the National Academies Report *Criteria for Selecting the Leading Health Indicators for Healthy People 2030* (released August 2019)

Finding 1: The committee finds that the *Healthy People 2030* draft objectives document is missing some key topics necessary to fully reflect the intent of the *Healthy People 2030* Framework's vision, mission, foundational principles, and overarching goals.

Finding 2: The committee finds that the draft objectives do not offer an appropriately balanced and comprehensive range from which to derive Leading Health Indicators (LHIs) that also reflect the intent of the *Healthy People 2030* Framework's vision, mission, foundational principles, and overarching goals.

Finding 3: The committee finds that the *Healthy People 2030* draft objectives document includes too few objectives that allow for making important comparisons to other countries, including to peer nations in the Organisation for Economic Co-operation and Development.

Finding 4: The committee finds that if the existing criteria for LHI selection were applied to the existing *Healthy People 2030* draft objectives, the resulting LHI set would not be aligned with the *Healthy People 2030* Framework—it would not tell a coherent story about the nation's (or communities') health, well-being, and state of health equity.

Recommendation 1: The committee recommends that the Department of Health and Human Services and the Federal Interagency Workgroup should add to the *Healthy People 2030* objectives topics or implement a structural reorganization (with additional topics) that will yield more core objectives that reflect the *Healthy People 2030* Framework and could lead to better LHIs. Cross-cutting topics (i.e., topics that refer to or link with multiple health states, life stages, systems, and all dimensions of health) should include health equity; the social, physical, and economic determinants of health; shared responsibility and multiple sectors; and all levels of government.

Recommendation 2: The committee recommends that a three-phase process should be used for LHI selection from the *Healthy People 2030* objectives. A new phase would precede the existing two, and it would apply the *Healthy People 2030* Framework (especially the vision, mission, foundational principles, and overarching goals) in consideration of additional objectives and in selecting LHIs.

MEASUREMENT LITERATURE REVIEWED

To prepare for the procedure that would yield a list of LHI contenders, the committee reviewed compilation of indicators prepared by study staff that were drawn from more than a dozen well-known and validated sets, including several that focused specifically on measures of health equity, or rather, measures of the factors that influence health equity. A brief overview of reviewed sets is provided in Table 2-2; note that this overlaps

TABLE 2-2 Select Measure Sets Reviewed by the Committee and Used as Reference for Identifying Candidate LHIs

	Reference Sets of Indicators					
Broad Topic or Domain for Which the Indicator Set Includes One or More Indicators	AHR	AHRQ Older Americans 2016	BARHII	CDC Winnable Battles	CHR	HHS HP2020
Length of Life	X	X			X	
Quality of Life		X			X	X
Tobacco	X	X		X	X	X
Nutrition, Physical Activity, Obesity	X	X		X	X	X
Alcohol/Substance Use	X		X		X	X
Sexual Health				X	X	
Access to Care	X	X	X		X	X
Quality of Care	X			X	X	X
Education		X	X		X	X
Employment		X	X		X	
Income	X	X	X		X	
Family/Social Support/Civic Engagement		X	X		X	
Community Safety	X		X	X	X	X
Environmental Quality	X	X	X		X	X
Housing, Transit		X	X		X	
Cost of Care/Medical Expenditures		X				

NOTES: The entries in this table are updated from the prepublication version of this report to more accurately reflect the content of these resources.
AHR = America's Health Rankings; AHRQ = Agency for Healthcare Research and Quality; BARHII = Bay Area Regional Health Inequities Indicators; CDC = Centers for Disease Control and Prevention; CHR = County Health Rankings; HHS HP2020 = Healthy People 2020

with but does not include all the measurement efforts presented at the May 28, 2019, information-gathering meeting (see agenda in Appendix B). The committee also reviewed measure sets or measurement efforts that focus primarily on tackling root causes of health disparities and advancing health equity, including the Bay Area Regional Health Inequities Indicators (BARHII), the HOPE Index, the National Equity Atlas, and the Prevention Institute Health Equity Indicators (BARHII, 2015; PolicyLink and USC PERE, 2018; Prevention Institute, 2015; Wong Croal et al., 2018).

HUD Healthy Communities Index	IOM HP2020	OECD Health at a Glance	OECD Social at a Glance	Prevention Institute Health Equity Indicators	IOM Vital Signs Report	WHO 100 Health Core	WIN
X	X	X	X		X	X	X
	X	X	X	X	X	X	X
	X	X	X	X	X	X	X
	X	X		X	X	X	X
X	X	X	X	X	X		X
	X			X	X	X	
	X	X		X	X	X	X
	X	X		X	X	X	
X				X	X		X
X			X	X			X
X		X	X	X			X
X			X	X	X		X
X	X		X	X		X	X
X	X			X		X	X
X			X	X			X
		X			X		

LHIs; HUD HCI = Department of Housing and Urban Development Healthy Communities Index; IOM HP2020 = 2011 IOM report on the HP2020 Leading Health Indicators; OECD = Organisation for Economic Co-operation and Development; Vital Signs = 2015 IOM Vital Signs report; WHO 100 Core = World Health Organization 100 Core Measures; WIN = Well-being in the Nation.

In addition to the key sets of metrics already listed here, and the information presented at the May 2019 meeting, the committee also reviewed some of the literature on measurement of health equity and the factors that shape it, and on well-being—two concepts that are central to the HP2030 Framework.

CONSIDERATIONS RELATED TO HEALTH EQUITY

The committee's thinking about measures to monitor equity was informed by the following list of Braveman's criteria:

- Indicators "must meet standard scientific and ethical criteria" (e.g., quality data and local knowledge).
- "[D]ifferences in the indicators between better- and worse-off groups should be relatively likely to reflect avoidable, unfair gaps in important conditions that could be narrowed through policy changes in any sector that influences health and not just health care."
- Appropriately disaggregated data "on the indicators is accessible for monitoring over time at the desired geographic level."
- "[I]ndicators must occur frequently enough in the groups to be monitored to permit reliable estimates of differences between the groups."
- [T]he range of indicators should include indicators of "health status, major determinants of health apart from health care, and key aspects of health care (e.g., financing, quality)." (Braveman, 1998, pp. 19–20)

The concept of *health equity* is related to *health disparity* and *health differences*. It is useful to briefly review these terms. Health differences refer to variations in rates of morbidity or mortality between two or more groups. There is no implication of any kind of causal reason for these variations. They are empirically observed differences. Health disparities, however, refer to health differences that are based on or originate in social disadvantages. A recent National Academies study defined health equity as "the state in which everyone has the opportunity to attain full health potential and no one is disadvantaged from achieving this potential because of social position or any other socially defined circumstance" (NASEM, 2017, p. 1). Braveman and colleagues offer the following definition that elaborates on socially defined circumstances:

> Health equity means that everyone has a fair and just opportunity to be as healthy as possible. This requires removing obstacles to health such as poverty, discrimination, and their consequences, including powerless-

> ness and lack of access to good jobs with fair pay, quality education and housing, safe environments, and health care. (Braveman et al., 2017, p. 2)

"[Ac]hieve health equity" is both part of a foundational principle and one of the five overarching goals of the HP2030 Framework.[2] Moreover, the framework's first foundational principle is "Health and well-being of all people and communities are essential to a thriving, equitable society." The committee interprets this framing (i.e., "all people and communities," and "equitable society") as reflecting a concern with the conditions that ensure "fair and just opportunity to be as healthy as possible" (Braveman et al., 2017). This suggests the importance not only of monitoring health data disaggregated by different demographic groups but also of monitoring the social and structural inequities that affect health.

The committee notes that the literature contains roughly four broad categories of measures relevant to health equity:

1. Traditional measures of health outcomes and health states (e.g., infant mortality rate, prevalence of diabetes) that are simply disaggregated by race, ethnicity, or other subpopulation; these shed light on disparities in health status and outcomes, but do not reveal causal pathways related to fairness or justice.
2. Measures of disparities in health care (e.g., colorectal screening, diagnosis, survival) that reveal some of the structural and systemic factors that shape the delivery, access, quality, and other aspects of care that contribute to unjustly disparate health outcomes (IOM, 2003; Mays et al., 2007).
3. Measures drawn from other sectors that shed light on factors that shape health outcomes (e.g., housing cost burden, access to transit or miles driven alone).
4. Measures that may themselves be shaped by underlying structural social inequities (e.g., segregation, redlining, unfair lending practices, bias in hiring), assessed by such measures as the Everyday Discrimination Scale and the Index of Dissimilarity (Shah et al., 2014).[3]

[2] See https://www.healthypeople.gov/2020/About-Healthy-People/Development-Healthy-People-2030/Framework (accessed February 12, 2019).

[3] For example, see the Boston Behavioral Risk Factor Surveillance System measure of "residence in public housing, subsidized housing, or neither" as a measure of inequities in the conditions that shape health and well-being, specifically, exposures to asthma triggers (see Shah et al., 2014). To compensate for the fact that the BRFSS sample "lacks power to conduct subgroup analyses in smaller neighborhoods," the Boston Public Health Commission "generates neighborhood and subgroup estimates by combining survey data from several years" (Shah et al., 2014, p. 2).

The committee noted that the first category—disaggregating key health indicators by race, ethnicity, and other demographics—has historically been a part of the Healthy People objectives and LHIs, but the committee agreed that in addition to continuing to providing disaggregated data for each LHI, the more robust focus on health equity reflected in the HP2030 Framework requires the addition of measures more explicitly linked with social equity and the creation of social, environmental, and economic conditions required for equitable health outcomes.

CONSIDERATIONS RELATED TO THE CONCEPT OF WELL-BEING

The World Health Organization (WHO) discusses well-being as existing "in two dimensions, subjective and objective. It comprises an individual's experience of their life as well as a comparison of life circumstances with social norms and values" (WHO, 2012). Well-being and health are seen as interactive concepts whereby health influences overall well-being, and well-being affects future health (WHO, 2012). The well-being construct was first introduced in the Healthy People initiative as part of HP2020, in the goal "Improve health-related quality of life and well-being for all individuals" (HealthyPeople.gov, 2019). The HP2020 website states the following:

> Promoting well-being emphasizes a person's physical, mental, and social resources and enhances protective factors and conditions that foster health. Instead of the traditional view of prevention as only avoiding or minimizing illness and risk factors, well-being also focuses on disease resistance, resilience, and self-management.

The SAC expanded the definition of well-being beyond the individual to acknowledge that it is an attribute of communities or society more broadly, and is shaped by a wide array of factors. The SAC's brief on "health and well-being" described the concept of well-being "as both a determinant and an outcome of health and reflects aspects of life that include physical, mental, emotional, social, financial, occupational, intellectual, and spiritual" factors (SAC, 2018b). The SAC further notes that health and well-being are mutually reinforcing, and importantly for communication and for appealing to stakeholders in other sectors, it asserts that well-being may be a "more motivating and unifying pursuit" than health (SAC, 2018b). The brief proposes that in the context of HP2030, "health and well-being can be defined as how people think, feel, and function" and also that there are "reciprocal influences between individual and societal health and well-being."

The Centers for Disease Control and Prevention (CDC) provides additional extensive discussion of well-being as part of its Health Related

Quality of Life (HRQOL) program. CDC describes measurement of well-being as including one's view of one's living conditions, "global judgments of life satisfaction from depression to joy," and "judging life positively and feeling good" (CDC, 2018).

The committee reviewed the draft core objectives for a measure of well-being, and finding none, it endeavored to identify and vet at least one to propose as an LHI. The committee has recommended a measure that is aligned with international measurement efforts (see below).

FIVE STEPS TO SELECT CANDIDATE LEADING HEALTH INDICATORS

Overview

The committee undertook two separate approaches resulting in five total steps in its effort to identify a slate of LHI candidates to recommend to the Department of Health and Human Services (HHS) (see Figure 2-1).

The terms top-down and bottom-up are intended to reflect the committee's consideration about the combination of approaches needed to identify a good working list of LHI candidates. "Top-down" refers to

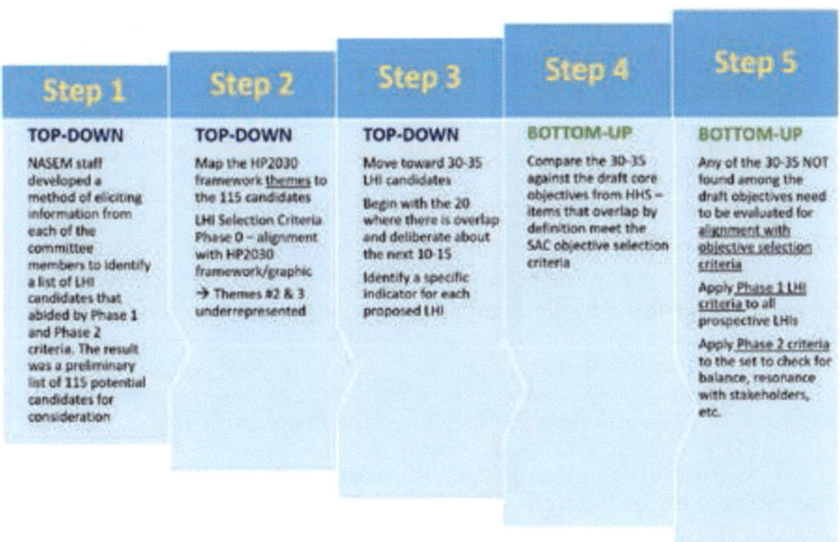

FIGURE 2-1 A graphic representation of the process undertaken by the committee to arrive at a list of Leading Health Indicators.

bringing the committee's combined expertise and judgment to bear on the selection of candidate LHIs, and "bottom-up" refers to the work of comparing the large number of existing draft HP2030 core objectives to the results of the top-down process to help identify LHI candidates. This step helped identify areas of overlap and gaps. The committee applied the objective selection criteria to committee-proposed LHI candidates not found on the HHS list of draft objectives to ensure that proposed measures qualified (see Box 2-1 for the objective selection criteria). Additionally, the final slate recommended to HHS would also need to adhere to the three categories of LHI selection criteria discussed in the first report (see Table 2-1). The committee also noted the importance of finding LHI measures useful to deploy at the state and local level, and LHI measures useful for making international comparisons.

The Top-Down Procedure

Committee members developed a list of potential indicators derived from more than a dozen sets of health metrics (see Table 2-2) that they identified as relevant to achieving the goal of selecting LHIs for HP2030. Using the curated list of resources as their primary reference, members were asked to identify candidates for consideration through the three-step top-down procedure (see Figure 2-1): (1) eliciting a set of 15 preferred priority indicators from each individual committee member; (2) mapping the resulting 115 candidates to the themes in the HP2030 Framework graphic; and (3) narrowing down the list of LHI candidates to 34—through a consensus process.

The Bottom-Up Procedure

There were roughly two steps for the bottom-up procedure: (1) approximately comparing the candidates resulting from the top-down procedure against the draft core objectives provided by HHS, and (2) applying the objective selection criteria to any items that were not found among current core objectives.

Reviewing the Evidence for Proposed LHIs

The committee considered the evidence for potential LHIs (and the objectives associated with them) at multiple points during the process. Evidence base is one of the criteria for selecting core objectives (see Box 2-1), and it specifies that the objective should have "a known evidence base, and identified evidence-based interventions to improve outcomes." The criterion calls for applying the evidence rating scale developed for HP2020: rigorous (4), strong (3), moderate (2), and weak (1).[4] Level 4 evidence is described as emerging from recommendations of the U.S. Preventive Services Task Force, the Community Preventive Services Task Force, or systematic reviews published in peer-reviewed journals. Level 3, or "strong" evidence, rests on nonsystematic reviews published by the federal government and nonsystematic reviews published in peer-reviewed journals. Level 2, seen as "moderate" evidence, emerges from journal articles of individual studies, published intervention research, and published pilot studies. Level 1, regarded as "weak," lists intervention evaluations or "studies without peer review that have evidence of effectiveness, feasibility, reach, sustainability, and transferability" (HHS, n.d.).

The committee recognizes the tension inherent in broadening the framework of considerations of health and well-being at the same time that HP2030 seeks to promote and adhere to high standards of evidence for intervention effectiveness. Measuring well-being implies drawing from a wider range of indicators, including some from outside the health sector, hence the potential for a wider range of types of interventions and evidence. It is the committee's view that in seeking LHIs that best represent high-level priorities for the nation, it will be important to maintain accommodation of levels of evidence appropriate to the domain, time frame, and type of intervention with respect to what constitutes evidence adequacy when drawing from work conducted in other sectors. This view resonates with the HP2020 publication *Evidence-Based Clinical and Public Health: Generating and Applying the Evidence*, which discusses the "limitations of the traditional hierarchy of evidence" and "the need for contextual information" (SAC, 2010, p. 11).

The evidence associated with potential LHIs is as varied as the LHIs themselves: some imply health care system interventions (e.g., contraceptives, HIV), others require "connecting the dots" to health outcomes (e.g., fourth grade reading proficiency), and others are endpoints to multiple pathways for intervention (e.g., life expectancy, infant mortality). This reality calls for articulating a different, broader, mental model for the relationship between LHIs and their evidence. LHIs are intended to move the dialogue and galvanize action by stakeholders; therefore, some indicators may not be supported by evidence that meets the criteria for "rigorous," but the perfect ought not to be the enemy of the good—less than perfect evidence may be warranted when there is a highly compelling reason to track a certain LHI. Moreover, the HP2030 effort centers well-being along with health and health equity, but markers of

[4] See HHS, n.d., or https://www.healthypeople.gov/2020/tools-resources/Evidence-Based-Resources (accessed May 5, 2019).

well-being do not necessarily have the same links to an evidence base that health measures do. The LHIs the committee proposes are supported either by evidence that specific interventions will improve outcomes or by evidence that the LHI is itself a marker of better health or well-being.

3

Details of the Top-Down Procedure

Drawing from more than a dozen sets of measures (for a complete version of the brief overview see Table 2-2) and in some cases, additional sources, committee members first generated a list of Leading Health Indicator (LHI) contenders based on each member's proposed indicators to inform the development of a high-level, parsimonious set. Two rounds of consolidating or collapsing similar items followed, and reduced the longer list of candidates to one that represented the committee's consensus of candidate LHIs.

In the process of selecting the first set of candidate LHIs for consideration, the top-down procedure employed a staff-developed, web-based polling form (developed using a web-based platform), which each member independently completed to ensure an efficient process and to avoid members influencing each other's thinking at an early stage. The form included a series of checks members were asked to make, reflecting key considerations required to ensure LHIs would adhere to all selection criteria and reflect *Healthy People 2030* (HP2030) principles. During this part of the work, committee members applied Phase 0 and Phase 1 LHI selection criteria to each LHI contender (see Table 2-1). For each candidate, committee members were asked to complete the following fields (see Appendix D for the form used):

a. Source of the suggested measure (e.g., America's Health Rankings, Centers for Disease Control and Prevention Winnable Battles)
b. Does the measure meet HP2030 objective criteria
c. Does the measure meet LHI selection criteria (Phase 0 and 1, with Phase 2 to be applied later to the full set; see Table 2-1)

d. Which of the four broad categories outlined in the committee's first report—life stages; public health and health care systems; social, physical, and economic determinants; or health states—does the measure fit in? The committee used this information as an additional way to ensure balance of measures
e. Which of the HP2030 Framework concepts (17 items; see Figure 1-1) does the measure map to?
   - **Health and Well-Being Across the Lifespan:** physical, mental, social dimensions of health; access to quality public health and clinical care systems (the committee separated the latter into four sub-level concepts: access to public health system, quality of public health system, access to health care, quality of health care) (seven items)
   - **Cultivating Healthier Environments:** physical, social, economic (three items)
   - **Closing Gaps:** health disparities, health equity, health literacy (three items)
   - **Increasing Knowledge and Action:** shared responsibility across sectors; public health successes; evidence-based laws, policies, and practices; objectives and data (four items)

Using the curated list of more than a dozen measure sets (see Table 2-2 for the high-level overview) each committee member was asked to identify 15 measures that would be eligible to be considered as a candidate LHI. The committee produced a pooled set of 115 LHI candidates. As foreseen, there were overlaps in LHI contenders produced by the committee, so the staff reviewed the list of 115 and condensed similar topics and measures, ultimately rendering a list of 45 distinct items. Next, the committee undertook a collective consensus process (several meetings discussing each LHI, alignment with selection criteria, and relevant literature) to further narrow the list, ultimately yielding the 34 LHIs presented in this report.

The resulting list of LHI candidates was heterogeneous, an assortment of complete measures (e.g., "life expectancy at birth"), broad topics with no specific measure (e.g., "education"), and multiple measures for the same topic listed together (e.g., for education, "either fourth grade reading proficiency or educational spending"). Staff collapsed the items submitted based on similarity, such as measures that were the same but worded differently or referred to the same topic, to yield a shorter list of 45 items.

The committee then deliberated in several rounds to arrive at consensus on the 34 LHI candidates to put forward. The committee arbitrarily considered that number would be appropriate in order to reflect the breadth of key priorities while advancing an achievable agenda toward health. At each step in the top-down process, the committee continually applied the three-phase LHI selection criteria (see Table 2-1), both explicitly during LHI selection (e.g., during the use of the polling tool) as well as throughout committee deliberations. Thus, the working assumption was that most candidates would meet the criteria. However, related considerations (e.g., "Does this LHI meet the 'public health burden' criterion?" and "What is known about interventions to address it?") operated throughout the deliberations, even before the committee moved on to the step of discussing the merits of each candidate LHI.

THE RESULTS OF THE TOP-DOWN PROCEDURE

As noted already, committee members were asked to contribute their suggestions toward a draft list of LHIs through a process that integrated a range of considerations and "checks." The result was a list of 34 LHIs, which are listed and discussed in the next chapter.

4

Results of the Bottom-Up Procedure: Gaps in the Draft Objectives

This chapter describes the bottom-up process of comparing the 34 Leading Health Indicator (LHI) candidates produced by the committee's top-down process (see Table 4-1) to the draft *Healthy People 2030* (HP2030) core objectives (see Appendix E) reviewed by the committee. The committee also consulted the seventh report of the Secretary's Advisory Committee on National Health Promotion and Disease Prevention Objectives for 2030 (SAC), containing that group's recommendations regarding objectives (SAC, 2019). The draft objectives had also been released to the public for comment during the months of December 2018 and January 2019, and the committee reviewed a summary of public comments received by the Department of Health and Human Services (HHS) in response to the *Federal Register* notice (NORC, 2019).[1]

LHIs DRAWN FROM EXISTING (DRAFT) HP2030 CORE OBJECTIVES

The committee found that 19 of its LHI candidates had draft HP2030 core objectives that matched the indicators committee members proposed (in Table 4-1, those are the items that include an acronym or abbreviation that represents the topic and the draft objective number, such as, SU-2030-03 Reduce drug overdose deaths, found under the topic heading "Substance Use" in the draft HP2030 objectives in Appendix E). The report

[1] This information is available from the National Academies Public Records Office at PARO@nas.edu.

TABLE 4-1 Recommended Leading Health Indicators, Specific Objectives, and *Healthy People 2030* Framework Concept with Which They Primarily Align

No.	LHI Candidate	Measure (new objective, unless HP2030 draft core objective is listed, denoted by XX-2030-XX*)	Themes[a]
1	Life expectancy	Increase life expectancy (at birth)	Closing Gaps: Health Equity
2	Child health	MICH-2030-02 Reduce the rate of all infant deaths	Health and Well-Being Across the Lifespan: Physical Health
3	Child health and well-being	Reduce the prevalence of one or more Adverse Childhood Experiences (ACEs) from birth to age 17	Health and Well-Being Across the Lifespan: Mental Health
4	Self-rated health	Increase the mean healthy days (CDC HRQOL–14 Healthy Days)	Health and Well-Being Across the Lifespan: Physical Health
5	Well-being	Increase proportion "thriving" on Cantril's Self-Anchored Striving Scale	Health and Well-Being Across the Lifespan: Physical Health
6	Disability	Reduce the percentage of adults aged 65 years and over with limitations in daily activities	Health and Well-Being Across the Lifespan: Physical Health
7	Mental disability	Reduce the rate of mental disability	Health and Well-Being Across the Lifespan: Mental Health
8	Substance use	SU-2030-03 Reduce drug overdose deaths	Health and Well-Being Across the Lifespan: Physical Health
9	Unintentional injury deaths	IVP-2030-03 Reduce unintentional injury deaths	Increasing Knowledge and Action: Physical Health
10	All cancer deaths	C-2030-01 Reduce the overall cancer death rate	Health and Well-Being Across the Lifespan: Physical Health
11	Suicide	MHMD-2030-01 Reduce the suicide rate	Health and Well-Being Across the Lifespan: Mental Health
12	Firearm-related mortality	IVP-2030-12 Reduce firearm-related deaths	Health and Well-Being Across the Lifespan: Physical Health
13	Maternal mortality rate	MICH-2030-04 Reduce maternal deaths	Closing Gaps: Health Equity

TABLE 4-1 Continued

No.	LHI Candidate	Measure (new objective, unless HP2030 draft core objective is listed, denoted by XX-2030-XX*)	Themes[a]
14	Mental health	Reduce percentage of adults who reported their mental health was not good on 14 or more days in the past 30 days (i.e., frequent mental distress)	Health and Well-Being Across the Lifespan: Mental Health
15	Oral health access	OH-2030-08 Increase the proportion of children, adolescents, and adults who use the oral health care system	Health and Well-Being Across the Lifespan: Physical Health
16	Reproductive health care services	FP-2030-07 Increase the proportion of sexually active adolescents aged 15 to 19 years who use any method of contraception at first intercourse	Health and Well-Being Across the Lifespan: Access to Quality Public Health and Clinical Care Systems
17	HIV incidence	HIV-2030-03 Reduce the number of new HIV diagnoses among persons of all ages	Health and Well-Being Across the Lifespan: Physical Health
18	Tobacco	TU-2030-13 Reduce use of any tobacco products by adolescents	Increasing Knowledge and Action: Evidence-Based Laws, Policies, and Practices
19	Obesity	NWS-2030-03 Reduce the proportion of children and adolescents aged 2 to 19 years who have obesity	Health and Well-Being Across the Lifespan: Physical Health
20	Alcohol use	SU-2030-13 Reduce the proportion of people with alcohol use disorder in the past year	Health and Well-Being Across the Lifespan: Physical Health
21	Immunization	Increase the proportion of 19–35-month-old children up to date on DTaP, MMR, polio, Hib, HepB, varicella, and pneumococcal conjugate vaccines	Increasing Knowledge and Action: Evidence-Based Laws, Policies, and Practices (also public health successes)
22	Hypertension rate	HDS-2030-04 Reduce the proportion of adults with hypertension	Health and Well-Being Across the Lifespan: Physical Health

continued

TABLE 4-1 Continued

No.	LHI Candidate	Measure (new objective, unless HP2030 draft core objective is listed, denoted by XX-2030-XX*)	Themes[a]
23	Ambulatory care-sensitive conditions/ avoidable hospitalization	Reduce discharges for ambulatory care-sensitive conditions per 1,000 Medicare enrollees (CMS-2)	Health and Well-Being Across the Lifespan: Access to Quality Public Health and Clinical Care Systems
24	Medical insurance coverage	AHS-2030-01 Increase the proportion of persons with medical insurance	Health and Well-Being Across the Lifespan: Access to Quality Public Health and Clinical Care Systems
25	Affordable housing	SDOH-2030-04 Reduce the proportion of all households that spend more than 30 percent of income on housing	Cultivating Healthier Environments: Social Environment
26	Environment	Improve the Environmental Quality Index	Cultivating Healthier Environments: Physical Environment
27	Environment	Lower the Heat Vulnerability Index	Cultivating Healthier Environments: Physical Health
28	Education	AH-2030-04 improve the fourth grade reading level	Cultivating Healthier Environments: Social Environment
29	Poverty	SDOH-2030-03 Reduce the proportion of persons living in poverty	Cultivating Healthier Environments: Economic Environment
30	Food security	NWS-2030-01 Reduce household food insecurity	Cultivating Healthier Environments: Social Environment
31	Civic engagement	Proportion of voting eligible population who voted in last election	Cultivating Healthier Environments: Social Environment
32	Social environment	Lower the Neighborhood Disinvestment Index	Closing Gaps: Health Equity
33	Social environment	Reduce the level of residential segregation captured by the Index of Dissimilarity	Closing Gaps: Health Equity

TABLE 4-1 Continued

No.	LHI Candidate	Measure (new objective, unless HP2030 draft core objective is listed, denoted by XX-2030-XX*)	Themes[a]
34	Social environment	Reduce the level of residential segregation captured by the Isolation Index	Closing Gaps: Health Equity

NOTE: DTaP = diphtheria; Hep B = hepatitis B; Hib = haemophilus influenzae type B; MMR = measles, mumps, rubella.

[a] Each candidate LHI may align with more than one of the themes in the HP2030 Framework graphic.

* Items that include an acronym or abbreviation that represents the topic and the draft objective number, such as "SU-2030-03: Reduce drug overdose deaths," are draft HP2030 objectives, which are listed in Appendix E. All others are new objectives.

does not provide any discussion about those LHIs, except for several cases that merit a brief comment. In the case of the measure for reproductive health care services, the committee would have preferred a broad measure of access for people of all genders, but it was unable to identify such a measure, so the objective FP-2030-07 ("FP" referring to the topic heading Family Planning) was a good option, given that it may shed some light on the issue of access and applies to all adolescents. In the case of the tobacco LHI, objective TU-2030-13 ("TU" for Tobacco Use), the committee believes this is appropriate for use as an LHI if "tobacco product" is a category that includes electronic nicotine delivery systems in addition to traditional cigarettes and other forms of tobacco.[2] Finally, in the case of the education-related LHI, the committee would have preferred an earlier life measure to the solid but chronologically "later" fourth grade reading proficiency measure, and the committee provides an explanation at the end of the chapter.

LHIs REQUIRING NEW CORE OBJECTIVES

Next, the committee discusses the LHIs proposed that do not have a corresponding objective. This responds to the part of the charge to the committee "to identify new objectives that meet the core objective criteria" (see Box 2-1 for the core objective selection criteria developed by the SAC). The committee also discusses gaps in and proposes new objectives to fill gaps in the draft

[2] The committee assumes that is the case because the data source listed for this objective is the Food and Drug Administration's National Youth Tobacco Survey (NYTS), and multiple sources discussing NYTS research, including Cullen et al. (2018) refer to e-cigarettes as a tobacco product.

core objectives and provides a justification for each, including whether or not each meets the HP2030 objectives criteria (see Box 2-1). The draft core objectives for HP2030 do not include some topics or measures that the committee considers important for consideration as LHIs. In some cases, a related objective was available in the draft core objectives, but the committee did not find it adequate to the task of serving as an LHI, for reasons such as a narrowness of focus. The committee lists the missing topics or objectives as follows:

1. Life expectancy
2. Child well-being
3. Self-rated health
4. Well-being
5. Physical disability
6. Cognitive disability or impairment (a broad measure)
7. Mental health (a broad measure)
8. Immunization (a broad measure)
9. Environmental exposure (a broad measure)
10. Climate change-related threats to health
11. Discharges for ambulatory care-sensitive conditions
12. Civic engagement
13. Social environment/health equity: a measure of residential segregation
14. Social environment/equity: a second measure of residential segregation
15. Social environment/equity: neighborhood-level disinvestment
16. Public health systems
17. Health care spending
18. Education (a measure of early childhood care and education)

The committee offers the following recommended LHIs. For three of the areas above, the committee was unable to find sufficiently robust objectives that met the objective selection criteria, finding instead that they were better suited for consideration as developmental objectives. These areas are an early childhood care and education measure; a measure of public health spending; and two measures of health care spending. The committee has made a finding in each of these areas.

For each new LHI it recommends (e.g., an LHI not based on an already existing HP2030 draft objective), the committee discusses (1) the current draft core objective(s) (if any) available on that topic and why existing objective(s) may not make good LHIs (i.e., too narrow or specific); (2) a reference to the HP2020 measures if appropriate to the context; (3) a brief summary of the literature about that measure (where else it is used, its research and validation); (4) how it meets objective selection criteria; and (5) how it meets LHI criteria.

Life Expectancy

The recommended objective statement for this LHI is: "Increase life expectancy at birth." The draft core objectives for HP2030 do not contain a life expectancy indicator. The committee recommends the LHI "increase life expectancy at birth." Life expectancy was a foundation measure of HP2020, it is a widely used and available measure at every level of government, and it is collected by the National Center for Health Statistics. Life expectancy is also important to track as an overall measure of the nation's health performance and as a means of comparing U.S. health to that of similar nations (OECD, 2017b)—as was acknowledged in HP2020 (HealthyPeople.gov, n.d.).

A life expectancy objective meets each of the objective selection criteria. It is a widely available and used measure, with ample current baseline data, it is of obvious national importance, and it is useful for assessing health equity and health disparities. The life expectancy objective has a known evidence base because there is deep knowledge about the factors that shape life expectancy. U.S. researchers and public health authorities have, for example, identified the key factors that contributed to an increase in life expectancy over the twentieth century, and they have similarly identified factors associated with an unprecedented decrease in life expectancy for some groups (particularly white, middle-aged men) in the second decade of the twenty-first century (see, for example, Case and Deaton, 2017).

Life expectancy may also be used to construct the Human Development Index (HDI) in combination with measures of educational attainment and a measure of per capita income (Measure of America, 2018; UNDP: Human Development Reports, n.d.). The HDI can be used for international comparisons, but as demonstrated by Measure of America, it may also be used at the state or local level for planning and tracking purposes.[3]

Life expectancy meets all LHI selection criteria: public health burden; magnitude of disparity (see, for example, Woolf et al., 2018); sentinel or bellwether (as noted above); and actionability—in the sense that life expectancy is a key indicator of society's ability to implement the range of evidence-based interventions needed to improve life expectancy.

Adverse Childhood Experiences

The recommended objective statement for this LHI is: "Reduce the prevalence of one or more adverse childhood experiences (ACEs) from birth to age 17."

Since 1998, when Felitti and his Kaiser Permanente colleagues published their research on ACEs (Felitti et al., 1998), the evidence has been accumulating about the lifelong effects on health and well-being of

[3] Lewis presentation, May 28, 2019.

adverse exposures (e.g., to abuse, severe deprivation) in childhood. National Academies reports *A Roadmap to Reducing Child Poverty* (NASEM, 2019a) and *Vibrant Healthy Kids: Aligning Science, Practice, and Policy to Advance Health Equity* (NASEM, 2019b) provide extensive discussion of the ways in which ACEs affect health and well-being later in life, and the latter also discusses the disparities along socioeconomic lines (e.g., children living in poverty are at greater risk of ACEs). Merrick et al. (2019) examined Behavioral Risk Factor Surveillance System (BRFSS) data from 25 states that collect state-added ACEs items and found that one in six adults reported having experienced four or more ACEs, and they found that ACEs were associated with multiple poor health outcomes. They concluded that interventions that prevent ACEs in childhood could reduce the prevalence of chronic conditions, risk behaviors, and other health outcomes in adulthood. Merrick et al. (2019) also noted that the Centers for Disease Control and Prevention's (CDC's) resource on ACEs provides evidence-based information about ways to prevent and mitigate exposure to ACEs (CDC, 2019). ACEs are also associated with increased likelihood of experiencing mental distress, substance use, and other health problems (see, for example, Bellis et al., 2019; Hughes et al., 2017).

Data on ACEs are available from multiple sources, and the measure available from the Health Resources and Services Administration's (HRSA's) National Survey of Children's Health (NSCH) is "prevalence of one or more Adverse Childhood Experiences from birth to age 17." The NSCH is funded and directed by HRSA and fielded by the U.S. Census Bureau.[4] Evidence of effective policy and programmatic interventions is being gathered by the National Child Traumatic Stress Network (NCTSN, n.d.). There is also a lot of work related to broader definition of ACEs and variation by income and race (see, for example, Mersky and Janczewski, 2018). CDC published *Preventing Adverse Childhood Experiences (ACEs): Leveraging the Best Available Evidence* (CDC, 2019), which offers a series of strategies and approaches for preventing ACEs, the latter ranging from implementing early childhood home visitation programming to strengthening household financial security.

Self-Rated Health

The recommended objective statement for this LHI is: "Increase the mean healthy days (CDC HRQOL–14 Healthy Days)." Although well-being is a core aspect of the HP2030 Framework and is paired with health (i.e., health and well-being) in each of the foundational principles in the

[4] This text has been revised since prepublication release.

framework, the draft core objectives for HP2030 do not include measures of well-being or a closely related construct used in HP2020—health-related quality of life (HRQOL). The committee recommends the CDC HRQOL–14 Healthy Days measure for use as an LHI. Such measures as the HRQOL–14, SF-36 (36-Item Short Form Survey), and SF-1 have been well-validated, with multiple studies showing "a statistically significant association between worse [general self-rated] health and a higher relative risk of mortality" (DeSalvo et al., 2006; Kaplan et al., 2017). A measure of self-rated health may be interpreted negatively or positively, and the committee suggests reporting on the full spectrum of responses, with positive and negative sides to allow framing that is appropriate to the use of the measure.

CDC HRQOL-14 Healthy Days meets all objective selection criteria. It is regularly collected as part of the BRFSS, and it could also be oversampled for some demographic groups. This measure also meets the following LHI Phase 1 criteria: public health burden and significance to health and well-being (as discussed earlier), magnitude of disparity (see Beck et al., 2014; CDC, 2008; Jones et al., 2008), and actionability.

Well-Being: Cantril Self-Anchoring Striving Scale

The recommended objective statement for this LHI is: "Increase the proportion of the population 'thriving' on Cantril's Self-Anchored Striving Scale." HP2020 described HRQOL and well-being as among the initiative's four overarching goals, as well as foundational measures. The concept of well-being is discussed as assessing "the positive aspects of a person's life, such as positive emotions and life satisfaction" and as "a relative state where one maximizes his or her physical, mental, and social functioning in the context of supportive environments to live a full, satisfying, and productive life."

Although self-rated physical and mental health were described as potential surrogates for HRQL, proposals for measuring well-being were described as "being explored." Given the centrality of the concept of well-being to the HP2030 Framework, the committee reviewed several self-reported approaches to capturing well-being. Although there has been wariness of using subjective measures based on a potential for relativism related to the expectations people attach to their circumstances, self-rated health has been found to be a better predictor of longevity than information about cardiovascular risk factors, including tobacco use, age, race, and years of education. Cantril's Self-Anchored Striving Scale, or the Cantril Scale, is a self-anchoring measure of well-being that has been used both nationally and internationally (OECD, 2011, 2017a). The measure asks people to rank well-being on a continuum from 0 (worst possible life) to 10 (best possible life) (Cantril, 1965). Scores of 7 and above are viewed as "thriving," those of 4 and below are described as "suffering," and intermediate scores where individuals have inconsistent well-being and double the sick days of the thriving are considered scores that denote "struggling." The scale is used for both the present and the future (5 years from now), and the two scales can be combined into an index.[5] The scale has been validated in multiple populations (e.g., children, different cultures) (Singh-Manoux et al., 2003), and as a quality-of-life indicator (OECD, 2013, 2017a; Singh-Manoux et al., 2003, 2005).

In a study of the impact of subjective social status, social determinants, and their association with ill health on working-age civil servants (n = 10,308), Singh-Manoux et al. (2003) found that subjective well-being, as captured by the Cantril Scale, was a predictor of ill health (i.e., angina, diabetes, respiratory illness, depression) separate from the conventional measures of socioeconomic position (education, income, and occupation). They suggest that a self-anchoring scale captures less well-defined sociocultural aspects of people's life circumstances that are critical to good health.

Helliwell et al. (2019) explored explanatory variables linked to national outcomes as measured by the Cantril Scale and found that gross domestic product (GDP) per capita, social support, healthy life expectancy, freedom to make life choices, generosity, and perceptions of corruption were predictors of a nation's ranking. The United States, with a score of 6.892 currently ranks 19th among developed nations (Helliwell et al., 2019). Data for the Cantril Scale are collected annually for the Gallup World Poll and the Gallup-Sharecare Well-Being Index (Gallup, n.d.) and capture well-being for OECD members.

The Cantril Scale is one of the Well-Being in the Nation measures proposed by the 100 Million Healthier Lives public–private partnership with the National Committee on Vital and Health Statistics, which advises the National Center on Health Statistics (100 Million Healthier Lives and the National Committee on Vital and Health Statistics, 2019).

One option to be considered in ensuring that data for this indicator, the Cantril Scale, are collected and accessible, is to add the question into a national survey, such as the BRFSS. This would help decision makers track well-being for U.S. subpopulations, with a focus on gaps to overcome to achieve equity.

This proposed well-being measure meets the following Phase 1 criteria for LHIs: public health burden, magnitude of disparity, bellwether.

---

[5] See https://news.gallup.com/poll/122453/understanding-gallup-uses-cantril-scale.aspx (accessed December 19, 2019).

Disability: Limitations in Daily Activities in Adults Aged 65 and Older

The recommended objective statement for this LHI is: "Reduce the percentage of adults aged 65 years and over with limitations in daily activities."

The HP2030 draft objectives contain six core objectives under the topic Disability and Health, but none is broad enough to serve as an LHI. The committee therefore recommends for use as an LHI: "Limitations in activities of daily living in adults aged 65 and older."

This measure meets the core objective selection criteria. It is measurable; a baseline is available along with additional data points (data regularly collected in the American Community Survey). This measure is of national importance, especially given the aging population and the need to understand future needs and implement programming to improve future outcomes, and there is a well-developed evidence base about the protective factors, such as being physically active (see van der Vorst, 2016). Regarding the fifth criterion for selecting core objectives (see Box 2-1), this measure also addresses health disparities and can inform efforts to support achieving health equity. Research from Fuller-Thomson et al. (2009) indicates that disparities in physical disability between black and white Americans are associated with differences in socioeconomic status (poverty and high school graduation); yet, even after adjusting for education level,

> race remained a significant predictor of functional limitations for men and women aged 55 to 64 and women aged 65 to 74 and of activities of daily living (ADLs) limitations for all race-age-gender groups.

Geronimus et al. (2006) have hypothesized that the repeated exposure to chronic stressors attributable to racism and discrimination causes more rapid deterioration in the health of African Americans. Geronimus et al. (2006) called this rapid aging "weathering" and stated the following:

> In the absence of a direct measure of weathering, investigators have studied diverse health indicators such as pregnancy outcome, excess mortality, and disability, and have found age patterns by race that are consistent with weathering. More broadly, scientists have sought to link bio-markers to social measures in an attempt to better understand the underlying physiological mechanisms of social disparities in health. (Geronimus et al., 2006, p. 263)

The measure Limitations in Activities of Daily Living in Adults 65 and Older meets the following LHI Phase 1 criteria: public health burden; relevance to addressing health disparities; and actionability.

Mental Disability (Cognitive Functioning)

The recommended objective statement for this LHI is: "Reduce the rate of mental disability." This measure from the U.S. Census ("Because of a physical, mental, or emotional condition lasting 6 months or more, the person has difficulty learning, remembering or concentrating") may be used as a general measure of cognitive disability in the population. Mental disability captures cognitive difficulties based on a wide range of conditions (e.g., genetic, traumatic, disease-related, psychiatric, dementia). Disaggregating its prevalence by different age cohorts allows the public and policy makers to understand the burden of disease and consider interventions to support individuals.

Cognitive impairment is a concern particularly as the population ages, and the committee did not find the three dementia-related core objectives adequate to consideration as an LHI.[6] Specifically, one measure, from the Health and Retirement Survey (DIA-2030-02) is too clinically oriented, and the other two measures are too indirect.

Although it is a somewhat heterogeneous measure in that it combines having "physical, mental, or emotional condition lasting 6 months or more" that produces "difficulty in learning, remembering or concentrating" this measure has the advantage of having easily accessible data for the entire country. The mental disability measure is not a measure of mental health in the population; rather it is a measure of cognitive disability in the population (which would include dementia, a condition that has a draft core objective associated with it).

The mental disability measure meets all objective selection criteria. The measure is available from the U.S. Census, includes both baseline and regularly updated data points, and can be disaggregated by race and ethnicity and other demographic groups. The measure also meets LHI Phase 0 criteria—specifically, it is relevant to the Health and Well-Being Across the Lifespan top-level concept of the HP2030 Framework (and as noted, especially for shedding light on an important dimension of the well-being of older adults), and it also meets Phase 1 selection criteria (public health burden; sentinel; actionable).

[6] DIA-2030-01 Increase the proportion of adults aged 65 years and older with diagnosed Alzheimer's disease and other dementias, or their caregiver, who are aware of the diagnosis; DIA-2030-02 Reduce the proportion of preventable hospitalizations in adults aged 65 years and older with diagnosed Alzheimer's disease and other dementias; DIA-2030-03 Increase the proportion of adults aged 65 years and older with Subjective Cognitive Decline (SCD) who have discussed their confusion or memory loss with a health care professional.

Mental Health: Frequent Mental Distress

The recommended objective statement for this LHI is: "Reduce percentage of adults who reported their mental health was not good in 14 or more days in the past 30 days (i.e., frequent mental distress)." The committee recommends this measure from the BRFSS, which assesses answers to the question "Now, thinking about your mental health, which includes stress, depression, and problems with emotions, for how many days during the past 30 days was your mental health not good?" This measure attempts to capture a broad range of mental health issues and is used in multiple well-known measurement sets, including the County Health Rankings.

The eight draft HP2030 core objectives do not include any general measures of mental health; the frequent mental distress measure could offer a measure that provides a broad sense of mental health in the population, at each level of measurement. This LHI also meets all objective selection criteria: it is measurable and both baseline data and additional data points are available from the BRFSS; it is of national importance; a robust evidence base exists for addressing mental distress (e.g., effectiveness of legislation promoting mental health benefits and integration of behavioral and primary care) (see Berry et al., 2017; Friedman et al., 2017); and the objective can help address equity and disparities if the data are disaggregated by race and ethnicity, among other demographic categories. This measure also meets Phase 1 LHI criteria: public health burden, serving as a sentinel or bellwether (given worsening mental health in some populations), and actionability.

Immunization

The recommended objective statement for this LHI is: "Increase the proportion of 19–35-month-old children who are up to date on DTaP, MMR, polio, Hib, HepB; varicella, and pneumococcal conjugate vaccines."

The draft core objectives for HP2030 include eight items that refer to vaccines and immunization, but none of those are sufficiently broad to warrant consideration for the LHIs. The committee recommends use of the measure "Children 19–35 months old who received recommended doses of diphtheria, tetanus and acellular pertussis (DTaP); measles, mumps and rubella (MMR); polio; Haemophilus influenzae type b (Hib); hepatitis B; varicella; and pneumococcal conjugate vaccines." This measure was an HP2020 LHI and one of the measures tracked annually by America's Health Rankings. Given its status as an HP2020 objective and LHI, it meets all relevant objective and LHI selection criteria, including being a potential bellwether for the status of acceptance of immunization as a safe and effective public health intervention and a sentinel for an upward trend in the prevalence of vaccine-preventable diseases.

Physical Environment: EQI

The recommended objective statement for this LHI is: "Improve the Environmental Quality Index (EQI)."

The HP2030 draft objectives contain 15 core objectives under the Environmental Health (EH) topic, ranging from "Reduce the number of days people are exposed to unhealthy air" (EH-2030-01) to "Increase the number of states, territories, tribes, and the District of Columbia that monitor diseases or conditions that can be caused by exposure to arsenic poisoning" (EH-2030-15). The core objectives available are largely related to broad environmental exposure (e.g., water or air, or to specific chemical exposure [e.g., lead, bisphenol A, perchlorate]). Only one objective is broader—EH-2030-07 Reduce the amount of toxic pollutants released into the environment, and would be a reasonable secondary candidate for LHI should the following recommendation not succeed.

For HP2030, the committee sought to find a comprehensive measure of environmental quality across the nation that is also available at the local level. The committee recommends the EQI as such a measure, which has been developed by the Environmental Protection Agency (EPA) and integrates data for five domains: air, water, land, built, and sociodemographic environments (Messer et al., 2014). A summary of its domains and the measures used to produce the index and the data sources are provided in Box 4-1.

Currently the EPA Office of Research and Development, National Health and Environmental Effects Research Laboratory (NHEERL), hosts publicly available data for the EQI for years 2000–2005. The data are available at the county level through EPA's Environmental Dataset Gateway.[7] A dataset for years 2006–2010 is expected to be publicly available in 2020, and a census track level EQI is under development.

Local, state, and national public health agencies as well as public health and environmental researchers at the county level can reproduce the EQI by using publicly available data. The methods for constructing and reproducing the EQI are available in the EQI Technical Report, and additional context is provided in peer-reviewed literature (Lobdell et al., 2011). A deep and growing evidence base assessing the relationship between environmental exposures captured by the EQI and their effects on health—mortality (Jian et al., 2017a,b) and morbidity (Gray et al., 2018a,b;

---

[7] See https://edg.epa.gov/data/Public/ORD/NHEERL/EQI (accessed November 21, 2019).

BOX 4-1
EPA's EQI (Environmental Quality Index): Domains, Measures, Sources

EQI Domain	Measure and Source
Air	1. Hazardous air pollutants (Air Quality System) 2. Hazardous air pollutant concentrations (National Emissions Inventory and meteorological data input into Assessment System for Population Exposure Nationwide)
Water	1. Water quality data (Watershed Assessment, Tracking, and Environmental Results Program Database/Reach Address Database) 2. National Contaminant Occurrence Database 3. Estimates of Water Use in the United States 4. Drought Monitor Data 5. National Atmospheric Deposition Program
Land	1. State-level pesticide usage (National Pesticide Use Database) 2. Measures of agricultural output (Census of Agriculture Full Report) 3. Indicators for major facilities (e.g., Superfund site) 4. Large quantity generators 5. Brownfield sites (EPA Geospatial Data Download Service)
Socio-demographic	1. County-level population and housing characteristics, including density, race, spatial distribution, education, socioeconomics, home and neighborhood features, and land use (U.S. Census) 2. County-level reports of violent crime (Uniform Crime Reports)
Built environment	1. Description of physical activity environment (recreation facilities, parks, physical fitness–related businesses), food environment (fast food restaurants, groceries, convenience stores), and education environment (schools, daycares, universities) per county (Dun and Bradstreet North American Industry Classification System codes) 2. Road type and length per county (Topologically Integrated Geographic Encoding and Referencing) 3. Annual pedestrian-related fatality per 100,000 population; maintained by National Highway Safety Commission (Fatality Annual Reporting System) 4. Housing authority profiles provide general housing details (low-rent and subsidized/section 8 housing); information updated by individual public housing agencies (Housing and Urban Development Data)

SOURCE: Abstracted from Lobdell et al., 2014.

Jagai et al., 2017; Rappazzo et al., 2015)—substantiates the index's utility as a sentinel for population health.

The EQI meets core objective selection criteria because environmental exposures are an established public health risk with the potential for mass exposures. Additionally there are well-documented health disparities in environmental risk exposures exerting an undue burden on marginalized populations (Lobdell et al., 2016) that merit equity considerations (Brulle and Pellow, 2006). The EQI's documented association with morbidity and mortality substantiates the index's utility as a sentinel or bellwether measure that is actionable at the county, state, and national levels.

Physical Environment: Heat Vulnerability Index

The recommended objective statement for this LHI is: "Lower the Heat Vulnerability Index."

The committee did not find any HP2030 draft core objectives that could be used to serve as a sentinel or bellwether related to climate change effects on health, but it was pleased to see the developmental objective "PREP-2030-D03 Increase the proportion of adults who are aware of their transportation support needs to evacuate in preparation of a hurricane, flood, or wildfire" under the "Preparedness" topic.

Because an LHI relevant to the health effects of climate change would be timely and important, the committee recommends the Heat Vulnerability Index (HVI) described by the Lancet Countdown on Health and Climate Change. The HVI can be derived from data in the Institute for Health Metrics and Evaluation Global Burden of Disease and is a measure of heat-related morbidity and mortality, including heat stress, cardiovascular disease, and renal stress. The committee first considered heat-related deaths, but ultimately concluded that the HVI may be more robust given its breadth.[8] The index ranges from 0 to 100 and is calculated using the

> mean of proportion of the population over 65 years; the prevalence of cardiovascular, diabetes and chronic respiratory diseases among population over 65 years using Global Burden of Disease study 2017 estimates; and the proportion of the population living in urban areas as a measure of exposure to urban heat island. (Watts et al., 2019)[9]

---

[8] EPA's technical documentation on heat-related deaths notes that "many deaths associated with extreme heat are not identified as such by the medical examiner and might not be correctly coded on the death certificate," leading to underestimating the heat-related mortality (EPA, 2017).

[9] See https://www.thelancet.com/cms/10.1016/S0140-6736(19)32596-6/attachment/7ec6fc0f-7b2f-4c9d-9c92-7cb88c875b59/mmc1.pdf (accessed November 25, 2019).

Broad overviews of health indicators related to climate change may be found in the federal government's Global Change Research Program Climate Change Assessment and in Ebi et al. (2018).

The effects of climate change on human health have been documented extensively; interventions to mitigate them are evolving, and many are well supported. Examples include emerging research on urban heat islands and ways to "cool" them through urban forestry; novel road, parking lot, and roofing materials; and other strategies. Several states and localities—San Francisco, New York State, Wisconsin, New York City, Philadelphia, to name a few—have developed or adapted an HVI to measure and improve their response to heat emergencies (see, for example, Madrigano et al., 2015; Wisconsin DHS, 2017). The committee notes that the HVI can be used for preparedness. Areas with a high HVI could use that information to prepare for and to prevent some of the mortality and morbidity (by deploying cooling centers, checking on isolated elders, etc.). The HVI's geography (urban) and demographics (aging populations) dimensions are actionable in the sense that they inform planning and preparation

The Lancet HVI meets objective selection criteria—it is a composite of several measurable items, and both baseline data and additional data points are available at the national level, and in many cases at the state, county, or local level. The measure also meets Phase 1 LHI selection criteria—the public health burden of climate change-associated health conditions has been growing, disparities are aligned with typical vulnerabilities (e.g., demographics, especially older age and along lines of race and ethnicity), and they typically layer over other disadvantages, such as economic and housing instability and poverty.

Health Care Quality: Discharges for Ambulatory Care-Sensitive Conditions

The recommended objective statement for this LHI is: "Reduce the discharges for ambulatory care-sensitive conditions per 1,000 Medicare enrollees (CMS-2)."

Over the past 25 years, ambulatory care-sensitive conditions (ACSCs) have been used at state, national, and international levels to track hospital discharges for illnesses that can be prevented through access to high-quality primary care. The committee recommends ACSCs as an LHI because of their ability to provide a picture of both access to and quality of ambulatory care delivery across the nation and regionally.[10] Hospitalizations

[10] See, for example, the Dartmouth Atlas, which allows users to view Medicare data on each Prevention Quality Indicator (PQI; see AHRQ, 2001) by state and different demographic categories.

for chronic conditions that could have been treated in outpatient settings mean that people experience unnecessary severity of illness, and health systems generate unnecessary cost. A study using data from the Medical Expenditure Panel Survey (2005–2010) reported that charges for ACSCs were four times higher when treated in inpatient rather than outpatient settings (Galarraga et al., 2015).

In 2011 ACSCs accounted for 10 percent of all hospitalizations and 5.8 percent of Medicaid inpatient stays (Stranges and Stocks, 2008). A large body of research has demonstrated that ACSC hospitalizations vary by income and by minority status, with higher rates of hospitalizations seen in African American and low-income populations (Billings et al., 1996; O'Neil et al., 2010). This disparity has raised questions about access to care (affordability and physical access) and differentials in quality of care provided. In reviewing the impact of Medicaid expansions under the Patient Protection and Affordable Care Act, Wen et al. (2019) report meaningful reductions in these hospitalizations.

The Agency for Healthcare Research and Quality (AHRQ) has selected 16 prevention quality indicators (PQIs) of ACSCs (AHRQ, 2001) culled from larger sets that are reliable and valid indicators that can be tracked through administrative data and are available at regional levels. These include conditions such as bacterial pneumonia, hypertension, dehydration, adult and pediatric asthma, urinary tract infections, chronic obstructive pulmonary disease, perforated appendix, and short and long-term complications of diabetes. The Centers for Medicare & Medicaid Services (CMS) has developed two composite measures based on Medicare data: an acute conditions composite (CMS-1) and a chronic conditions composite (CMS-2) (CMS, 2015). CMS-2 could be used as the LHI for ACSCs, revealing crucial insights about the functioning of the health care delivery system and about unnecessary costs that compound the overarching problem of out-of-control health care costs. Medicaid data could also be mined for ACSCs, as those data are likely available at state and national levels for younger (non-Medicare) populations, where avoidable hospitalizations are particularly problematic.

The composite ACSC measure CMS-2 meets the objective and LHI (Phase 1) selection criteria.

Social Environment: Civic Engagement—Voter Participation

The recommended objective statement for this LHI is: "Increase the proportion of voting-eligible population who votes."

The committee believes that because dimensions of social capital (i.e., civic engagement and social cohesion) have implications for health, it is important to consider them in composing the set of LHIs. There is a large literature on social capital, some of which has been previously reviewed as part of the Healthy People work.[11] Committee members considered several possible measures of social capital and came to agree with those who have incorporated a measure of civic engagement in indicator sets—that people's interest in creating and sustaining a vibrant polity and social fabric appears to be associated with other measures of well-being. Although some measures of social capital may not be sufficiently robust, whether due to a not yet adequate evidence base or other issues, such as difficulties measuring in subpopulation or other data challenges, voting participation appears to be a reasonably strong measure (see, for example, NRC, 2014).

The Well-being in the Nation measure set lists "total votes cast in the most recent midterm or presidential election as share of total voting-age citizens." The Robert Wood Johnson Foundation (RWJF) Culture of Health measures also include voting participation, as does America's Health Rankings, and the Department of Housing and Urban Development (HUD) Healthy Communities Index, which uses "proportion of voting-eligible population who voted in last election."

Voting is a way to operationalize social capital. Murayama et al. (2012) conducted a review that found "both individual social capital and area/workplace social capital had positive effects on health outcomes," but they noted that more research was needed to show how building social capital can improve health (Murayama et al., 2012). Evidence of the relationship between voting and health indicates it is bi-directional, and historically, there has been more research showing health status affects voting behavior (Blakely et al., 2001; Denny and Doyle, 2007; Reichel, 2018). Some evidence of the positive effects that voting participation has on health has been emerging in recent years. Research from Klar and Kasser (2009)—cited in support of the RWJF voting participation measure—had shown that "several indicators of activism were positively associated with measures of hedonic, eudaimonic, and social well-being" (Klar and Kasser, 2009). A study by Ballard et al. (2019) shows a positive association between voting and volunteerism behaviors in adolescence and positive health effects in later life, including better mental health and lower likelihood to engage in unhealthy behavior. Panel studies using Canada's General Social Survey to assess the effect of three dimensions of social capital (social networks and social support, civic participation, and social participation) on self-rated health have shown causation in both directions (Habibov and Weaver, 2014). Two additional studies that examined the relationship between

[11] See https://www.healthypeople.gov/2020/topics-objectives/topic/social-determinants-health/interventions-resources/social-cohesion (accessed December 9, 2019) and also https://www.healthypeople.gov/2020/topics-objectives/topic/social-determinants-health/interventions-resources/civic-participation (accessed December 9, 2019).

Medicaid expansion and voter participation have shown at least a temporary positive relationship (Clinton and Sances, 2018; Haselswerdt, 2017).

The proposed voter participation LHI meets all objective selection criteria: it is measurable and has both baseline and additional data points (U.S. Census Current Population Survey; see also NRC, 2014), the evidence base for it is fairly strong and growing, and it has considerable bearing on health equity and disparities given the robust understanding of what shapes structural inequities (NASEM, 2017). Voter participation is a measure of national importance for several reasons.[12] Voting is a reflection of social capital, and the relationship between social capital and health is well established (Ehsan, 2019; Murayama et al., 2012). This is noteworthy, along with the growing evidence linking voting with health. It is, however, important to view voting participation in its broader context, which includes an understanding of voting administrative burdens and potential voter suppression, along with disenfranchisement experienced by people with involvement in the criminal justice system, and individuals experiencing housing instability. These factors demonstrate a key weakness of voting participation—the variation in the denominator from one state to another, depending on the array of laws, policies, and practices that shape voting behavior and voting access.

Equity: Neighborhood Disinvestment Index

The recommended objective statement for this LHI is: "Lower the Neighborhood Disinvestment Index."

The index is a measure pertinent to structural inequity. It is a measure included in the Prevention Institute health equity measures, and it includes such standardized data collection of the following:

1. Percent of residents in poverty
2. Percent of (male) unemployed residents
3. Percent home ownership (or some other measure of residential stability such as average length of current residence)
4. Percent single parent/single income households
5. Percent of residents with low educational attainment (and/or the reverse, percent residents with college degrees)
6. Percent of residents in management/professional occupations (sometimes the age structure and/or the racial/ethnic composition of the neighborhood is also included)

---

[12] Described in the Objective Selection Criteria for Core Objectives as having "a direct impact or influence on health, broad and comprehensive applicability, a substantial burden," and "address a national health priority."

Poverty, low educational attainment, and the lack of opportunity are powerful influences on health and well-being (see, for example, Chetty and Hendren, 2017; Chetty et al., 2016; NASEM, 2017, 2019a,b), and the committee underscores the importance of monitoring poverty as part of its efforts to improve population health by addressing the social and structural factors that shape health and equity.

The Neighborhood Disinvestment Index meets the criteria for core objective selection. It is measurable, constructed from existing U.S. Census data for which both baseline and additional data points are available; it is of national importance (health impact, broad applicability, substantial burden, and a national public health priority); it is based on rigorous evidence for each component of the index (see, for example, Chetty and Hendren, 2017; Izenberg et al., 2018; Pickett and Pearl, 2001; Sampson et al., 2002); and it is highly relevant to health equity and disparities.

Equity: Residential Segregation (Two Measures)

The recommended objective statements for this LHI are: "Reduce the level of residential segregation captured by the Index of Dissimilarity; and Reduce the level of residential segregation captured by the Isolation Index."

As noted earlier, the draft core objectives lack measures of equity that shed light on the causes of health disparities (i.e., structural inequities). The committee recommends the LHI racial and ethnic residential segregation, drawing two measures that can be easily calculated with data collected by the U.S. Census, the Index of Dissimilarity, and the Isolation Index (Iceland et al., 2002; Massey and Denton, 1993; Weinberg et al., 2002). Segregation has been considered a key determinant of racial/ethnic inequities in health (Gee and Payne-Sturges, 2004; Mehra et al., 2017; Williams and Collins, 2001).

The committee recommends two LHIs that capture racial and ethnic residential segregation, the Index of Dissimilarity and the Isolation Index. Both are commonly used measures in the literature, they capture two different dimensions of residential segregation (Massey and Denton, 1993), and some studies show that they do not have equivalent associations with health outcomes or health risk factors (Goodman et al., 2018; Kramer and Hogue, 2009; Nobles et al., 2017).

The Index of Dissimilarity and the Isolation Index can be calculated using the data from the U.S. Census. The former measures how evenly racial and ethnic groups are distributed across geographic areas, whereas the latter captures the degree to which one racial/ethnic group might have contact with other racial or ethnic groups. Dissimilarity has been linked to the unequal distribution of local and municipal resources, as well as exposure to environmental toxins (LaVeist et al., 2011; Morello-Frosh and Jesdale, 2006;

The Annie E. Casey Foundation 2019). Isolation has been linked to problems such as restricted access to health care facilities and to transmission of infectious diseases (Acevedo-Garcia, 2000; Dai, 2010). For example, Hayanga et al. (2009) found that in counties with high rates of isolation segregation were related to lower access to surgical services among minority populations, compared to counties with less segregation. The 2019 County Health Rankings report shows that higher levels of residential segregation are associated with higher rates of severe housing cost burden for households headed both by whites and by blacks, demonstrating that inequity can have widespread effects (County Health Rankings and Roadmaps, 2019).

It is increasingly recognized by multiple sectors that racial residential segregation is an important determinant of social, economic, and health-related well-being (County Health Rankings & Roadmaps Program, 2019; HUD, 2015; Landrine et al., 2017). Chetty et al. (2019) have found that neighborhood-level segregation affects economic opportunity. Segregation has been considered a key determinant of racial and ethnic inequities in health (Gee and Payne-Sturges, 2007; Mehra et al., 2017; Williams and Collins, 1999). For example, data from the Coronary Artery Risk Development in Young Adults (CARDIA) study showed that changes in segregation were associated with changes in systolic blood pressure over 25 years (Kershaw et al., 2017).

The committee discussed both community or structural and individual-level measures of discrimination, like the Everyday Discrimination Scale, or the BRFSS Reactions to Race measure that is included in the Well-being in the Nation measure set (100 Million Healthier Lives and NCVHS, 2019), but ultimately concluded that a structural and/or community-level measure would be more useful as an LHI.

The measures of residential segregation meet core objective selection criteria: measurable, with baseline data and two additional data points; of national importance, with robust evidence on the relationship between segregation and well-being and health; and of great relevance to addressing disparities and improving health equity. The measures also meet LHI selection criteria (measurable; both baseline and other data points are available from the U.S. Census; there is robust evidence that mitigating residential segregation can lead to improved well-being and thus health [Chetty and Hendren, 2017]; and it is actionable).

DISCUSSION OF LHI OBJECTIVES PARTLY FOUND AMONG THE HP2030 DRAFT CORE OBJECTIVES

The following three topics and corresponding LHI contenders were found among the HP2030 draft core objectives but deserve additional discussion. These are the objectives on tobacco, poverty, and education.

Adolescent Use of Tobacco Products

The recommended objective statement for this LHI is: "Reduce current use of any tobacco products among adolescents (TU-2030-03)." The committee would clarify the meaning of the term "tobacco products." If the objective is intended to include electronic nicotine delivery systems, the committee agrees that it is adequate to serve as a Leading Health Indicator. Both CDC (in BRFSS) and the Food and Drug Administration (in the National Youth Tobacco Survey) use the term "tobacco products" to refer to all types of cigarettes, including electronic, along with other products (such as chewing tobacco).

Poverty

The recommended objective statement for this LHI is: "Reduce the proportion of persons living in poverty (SDOH-2030-03)."

The committee recommends disaggregating this by age group, with particular attention to child poverty. The committee notes, as did the SAC, that child poverty is essential to track because of the implications it has for health and well-being in later life (see, for example, Chetty et al., 2016). The core objective SDOH-2030-03 "Reduce the proportion of persons living in poverty" meets core objective selection criteria, and so does child poverty, but the committee would like to underscore the robust evidence base that links child poverty with a range of poor health outcomes, extensively discussed and documented in two recent National Academies reports on child health and well-being (NASEM, 2019b) and on child poverty (NASEM, 2019a). The 2019 report *A Roadmap to Reducing Child Poverty* found that "many programs that alleviate poverty—either directly, by providing income transfers, or indirectly, by providing food, housing, or medical care—have been shown to improve child well-being" (NASEM, 2019a). The same report listed the Earned Income Tax Credit Program and improvements in child educational and health outcomes; the Supplemental Nutrition Assistance Program (SNAP) and improved "birth outcomes as well as many important child and adult health outcomes"; and "expansions of public health insurance for pregnant women, infants, and children" that "have led to substantial improvements in child and adult health, educational attainment, employment, and earnings" (NASEM, 2019a).

Social Environment: Education

The recommended objective statement for this LHI is: "Improve fourth grade reading level (AH-2030-04)." The committee believes that including an LHI on education is crucial given the extensive evidence on the relationship between educational attainment and health status in later life (NASEM, 2019b; NRC and IOM, 2013; Woolf et al., 2007). Although educational attainment is a protective factor and has a positive relationship with health, the magnitude of the benefit reaped by different sociodemographic groups is disparate/unequal. The committee recommends as an LHI related to education "Increase the proportion of fourth grade students whose reading skills are at or above the proficient achievement level for their grade" (AH-2030-04 in the draft HP2030 core objectives). This measure is supported by evidence indicating that children who are not proficient in reading at the start of fourth grade face a greater likelihood of high school dropout and associated lower earning potential (Hernandez, 2012), and school dropout is associated with poorer social and health outcomes (Lansford et al., 2016).[13] The committee would have preferred an early childhood education measure, but as discussed below, the measure it sought is not available at this time.

CONSIDERATIONS FOR POTENTIAL DEVELOPMENTAL OBJECTIVES

A Developmental Objective for Early Childhood Care and Education

The HP2030 draft core objectives contain several good options: fourth grade reading proficiency, chronic school absence, and on-time high school graduation. (It is important to note that these measures reflect system-level failure or success and should not be interpreted as simply measures of individual effort or capability.) Although the committee selected fourth grade reading proficiency as an LHI because of its importance to academic achievement later in life (The Annie E. Casey Foundation, 2013), the committee would have preferred a measure for tracking earlier-life educational experiences, such as access to quality early childhood care and education. Quality early childhood care and education are key to school success (NASEM, 2019b), but the committee was unable to find an adequate measure, apart from the measure "3- and 4-year olds in school" as an LHI as the next best thing.

The Administration for Children and Families (ACF) in HHS has several relevant resources. Its report *Defining and Measuring Access to High-Quality Early Care and Education: A Guidebook for Policymakers and Researchers* discusses measurement, but it does not provide a national-level measure of early childhood care and education quality. The Quality Rating and Improvement System (QRIS) approach developed by ACF offers states

[13] Note that the literature includes measures of third as well as fourth grade reading proficiency.

guidance, resources, and some funding to implement QRISs for early- and school-age care and education programs. Although many states have QRISs, there is no national system of measurement, and it is up to the states how they implement the standards (NASEM, 2019b). Validation of the QRIS approach is mixed and it is largely a point of entry to promote high quality programming and is not broadly or uniformly adopted by states (NASEM, 2019b). Moreover, "[t]he difference in [QRIS] system designs across states make it difficult to draw general conclusions from these validation studies about their links to various domains of children's development, especially health. The voluntary nature of QRISs in most states and the varying standards also make it difficult to establish a causal link between them and child outcomes" (p. 392). From the standpoint of equity, although states could and many do rate early childhood education programs (public or private), there is also a concern about ratings potentially victim-blaming under-resourced school systems or communities.

The Annie E. Casey Foundation, which produces the annual *Kids Count Data Book,* includes the following four education measures: young children ages 3 and 4 not in school, fourth graders not proficient in reading, eighth graders not proficient in math, and high school students not graduating on time. Although the discussion of the first measure (enrollment in early childhood education) acknowledges the importance of high quality programs, the measure itself is merely a measure of access, not access to quality services (The Annie E. Casey Foundation, 2019).

The *Kids Count Data Book* states the following:

> Although Head Start and the expansion of state-funded programs since the 1990s have greatly increased access to preschool and kindergarten, many kids—especially 3-year-olds and children living in low-income families—continued to be left out, exacerbating socioeconomic differences in educational achievement. Among member countries of the Organization for Economic Cooperation and Development, the United States has the third-lowest percentage of young children enrolled in early childhood programs. (The Annie E. Casey Foundation, 2019, p. 30)

The *Data Book* reports that during 2015–2017, 52 percent of U.S. children ages 3 and 4 (4.2M) were not in school (The Annie E. Casey Foundation, 2019). The committee found that although (1) there are measures of access to preschool (or pre-kindergarten, or early childhood care and education program), (2) there is evidence that quality early childhood care and education are crucial, and (3) there are no measures of access to quality early childhood care and education. In the absence of a measure of access to quality early childhood care and education—an important predictor of educational and other outcomes, the committee made the following finding:

The committee finds that a developmental objective of access to quality early childhood care and education could draw attention to the importance of starting early in placing children on the pathway to fourth grade reading proficiency and other measures of educational success.

Costs and Investments in Public Health and Health Care

The Cost of Health Care

The committee was in full agreement that the high cost together with the poor distribution of medical care—where some families and individuals lack access to needed care—is a significant impediment on the economic stability of Americans and the national economy (Auerbach and Kellermann, 2011; Baicker, 2001; Orszag and Kane, 2003). Research indicates that states offset the Medicaid increases with less support for other programs targeting lower-income residents, and health care cost growth harms the economy with repercussions for American families. There is an opportunity cost of foregoing social goods that have been shown to be greater correlates of population health (higher education), as those social goods have become increasingly unaffordable because of health care budgets—Orszag and Kane (2003) have shown that rising Medicaid costs negatively affect state university system funding.

At the same time that health care costs continue to rise, many members of the public continue to be uninsured or underinsured, thereby making needed medical care inaccessible. Per capita health care costs in the United States are far greater than those of peer nations, and yet U.S. health outcomes remain disappointing when compared internationally (NRC and IOM, 2013; OECD, 2017). Accordingly, the committee initially considered setting targets for reductions in per capita health care spending as an LHI. However, since aggregate spending measures are minimally informative about the extent of overtreatment (spending too much without health benefits), undertreatment (spending too little for effective care), or excess prices relative to other high-income countries, the committee concluded that tracking per capita expenditures alone would not be sufficient.

Instead of recommending an LHI of per capita or percent GDP health care expenditures, the committee discussed tracking the cost of a market basket of widely used pharmaceuticals in comparison to their cost in other affluent nations as a next best measure relevant to health care spending. There is evidence that the high price of U.S. pharmaceuticals has led many patients to reduce their use of potentially life-saving drugs (Borrescio-Higa, 2015); this in turn is likely to adversely affect health. Thus, the committee viewed as desirable the objective of tracking the cost of U.S. pharmaceuticals in comparison to other high-income nations, where greater alignment with these countries is viewed as a positive development. The high price of U.S. pharmaceuticals has rendered them unaffordable to many individuals with chronic and life-threating diseases (Cohen et al., 2019) and continues to take a toll on people's health. Tracking the cost of U.S. pharmaceuticals in an international perspective is aligned with the HHS objective to make U.S. pharmaceuticals comparably priced to other nations, so

> the committee finds that a developmental objective that tracks the cost of a "market basket" of widely used pharmaceuticals in comparison to their cost in other affluent nations could be informative to multiple stakeholders.

The 2018 HHS study Comparison of U.S. and International Prices for Top Medicare Part B Drugs by Total Expenditures highlights current thinking in the department about the rationale for addressing the fact that costs for top drugs under Medicare Part B are 1.8 times higher than those of other countries (ASPE, 2018).[14]

Administrative Costs

This is another subset of health care spending that warrants attention. Considerable research has repeatedly indicated that a large proportion of health care spending, perhaps as much as 30 percent, is wasted (IOM, 2006), and administrative costs are one of the drivers (Anderson et al., 2019). A Commonwealth Fund study found that in the United States, the 2015 cost of health insurance administration was $787, compared to just under the $100 OECD median, and $89 for Sweden, $90 for the United Kingdom, and $141 for Canada (Tikkanen, 2018). The United States does not measure this routinely, possibly because there is no consensus on a measure that would be adequate to the task. Given the evidence of a stunning difference in administrative (and overall) spending between the United States and peer nations, and juxtaposed with the nation's lackluster health performance, the committee believes that an actionable administrative cost measure that is not linked with any political agenda could be a useful and compelling indicator. Therefore the committee made the following finding:

The committee finds that a developmental objective on health care system administrative cost could provide a concrete proxy for health

---

[14] See https://aspe.hhs.gov/pdf-report/comparison-us-and-international-prices-top-medicare-part-b-drugs-total-expenditures (accessed December 20, 2019).

care spending more broadly, and could offer compelling and easier to communicate information to a range of audiences.

Public Health Spending

The HP2030 core draft objectives contain seven items under the topic Public Health Infrastructure (and an additional seven developmental objectives). The committee did not find any of the draft objectives well suited to serving as an LHI either because they are narrow or because—although accreditation and its effects on quality are important—insufficient evidence is available to link aspects of public health system quality with health outcomes. Measures of public health accreditation are important, but they may be solely indicative of public health system ability to perform at a higher level (Riley et al., 2012).

Public health expenditure as a proportion of total health spending has declined to levels not seen since the Great Depression (Himmelstein and Woolhandler, 2016). In 2017, the United States spent $88.9 billion on government public health activities out of $3.49 trillion (CMS.gov, 2018; Martin et al., 2019). Public health expenditure currently accounts for less than 5 percent of U.S. spending (Sensenig, 2007; TFAH, 2006), and it is projected to decline to 2.4 percent by 2023 (Himmelstein and Woolhandler, 2016). The decrease in funding seems unjustified as the evidence of positive returns on investments in public health continues to accumulate (Brown, 2016; Mays and Smith, 2011; McCullough, 2019). Internationally, a systematic review of the return on investment on public health interventions in high-income countries, which included 52 peer-reviewed studies, estimated that the overall median return on investment (ROI) for public health interventions is 14.3 to 1 (Masters et al., 2017). Stratifying the interventions by geographic location showed that for local public health interventions the median ROI was 4.1 to 1, and for nationwide public health interventions, the median ROI was 27.2 to 1. The conclusion was that local and national public health interventions are highly cost-saving and that therefore disinvestments in public health interventions are a "false economy" because these decrements induce additional costs to health care services and the economy in general. In terms of morbidity, research has shown that public health investments yield results for specific outcomes (Singh, 2014). Other research has found that public health staffing and the provision of maternal and child services have a positive effect on infant health (Schenck et al., 2015), and state-level public health spending is associated with lower rates of certain vaccine-preventable diseases in subsequent years (Verma et al., 2017). In terms of mortality, studies have documented a decrease in preventable deaths (infant mortality, cardiovascular disease deaths, diabetes, and cancer) (Mays and Smith, 2011) and in all-cause mortality (Leider et al., 2018). The hypothesized/plausible mediating mechanism, that is, the link between improved funding and better population health outcomes, seems to be the improved organizational capacity of public health agencies to improve internal processes and performance, which ultimately influence outcomes (Handler et al., 2001; Meyer et al., 2012; Scutchfield et al., 2009). Mays and Mamaril (2017) also found that public health expenditures offset Medicare expenditures.

The committee believes that public health spending is a more promising measure than other indicators related to access to and quality of public health services, but the wide variation in how public health funding is allocated, distributed, and reported limits the reliability of the data somewhat. Public health funding data include administrative data available from the CMS Office of the Actuary in the U.S. Census Bureau's Census of State Governments and survey data from the Association of State and Territorial Health Officials' Profile of State and Territorial Public Health. The measure also meets LHI Phase 1 selection criteria: addresses a public health burden, may be a sentinel given association between drops in public health funding and health status, and is actionable (see, for example, IOM, 2012). Therefore the committee made the following finding:

> The committee finds that the developmental objective per capita public health funding would elevate the profile of an often overlooked component of "health spending" writ large, and given the growing research and attention to data challenges, the measure's reliability and validity will likely be confirmed over the coming decade.

Comparison to HP2020 LHIs

The committee compared the recommended set of HP2030 LHIs to HP2020 LHIs and found both a great deal of congruence and some differences that highlight the newly proposed set's alignment with the components of the HP2030 Framework and in particular the attention to well-being, health equity, and the role of partners in non-health sectors (see Table 4-1). These differences have yielded an LHI set that is distributed across several more topics (general health/well-being/health-related quality of life; determinants of health equity; more social determinants, including a separate topic for social capital and specifically the civic engagement domain). The topics in the left column of Table 4-2 are provided in alphabetical order (per the HHS HP2020 website), and the topics on the right were slotted in partially alphabetical order, unless it was not possible to do so, such as in the case of topics closely related to HP2020 topics.

TABLE 4-2 Side-by-Side Comparison of *Healthy People 2020* Leading Health Indicators and Recommended *Healthy People 2030* Leading Health Indicators

HP2020 LHIs	Recommended HP2030 LHIs
Access to Health Services	Access to Health Services
• Persons with medical insurance (AHS-1.1)	AHS-2030-01 Increase the proportion of persons with medical insurance
• Persons with a usual primary care provider (AHS-3)	
	Health Care System Quality
	• Discharges for ambulatory care-sensitive conditions
	Health Care Access
Clinical Preventive Services	Clinical Preventive Services
• Adults receiving colorectal cancer screening based on the most recent guidelines (C-16)	
• Adults with hypertension whose blood pressure is under control (HDS-12)	• HDS-2030-04 Reduce the proportion of adults with hypertension
• Persons with diagnosed diabetes whose A1c value is greater than 9 percent (D-5.1)	
• Children receiving the recommended doses of DTaP, polio, MMR, Hib, HepB, varicella, and PCV vaccines by age 19–35 months (IID-8)	• Children receiving the recommended doses of DTaP, polio, MMR, Hib, HepB, varicella, and PCV vaccines by age 19–35 months
	Determinants of Health Equity
	• Neighborhood Disinvestment Index
	• Residential Segregation: Index of Dissimilarity
	• Residential Segregation: Isolation Index
Environmental Quality	Environmental Quality
• Air Quality Index >100 (EH-1)	• Environmental Quality Index
• Children exposed to secondhand smoke (TU-11.1)	• Heat Vulnerability Index

TABLE 4-2 Continued

HP2020 LHIs	Recommended HP2030 LHIs
	General health, health-related quality of life, well-being
	• Life expectancy at birth
	• CDC HRQOL-14 (healthy days)
	• Cantril Scale
	• Limitations in daily activities in adults aged 65 and older
	• Mental disability
	• Prevalence of adverse childhood experiences
Injury and Violence	Injury
• Injury deaths (IVP-1.1)	• IVP-2030-12 Reduce firearm-related deaths • IVP-2030-03 Reduce unintentional injury deaths
• Homicides (IVP-29)	
Maternal, Infant, and Child Health	Maternal, Infant, and Child Health
• All Infant deaths (MICH-1.3)	• MICH-2030-02 Reduce the rate of all infant deaths
• Total preterm live births (MICH-9.1)	• MICH-2030-04 Reduce maternal deaths
Mental Health	Mental Health
• Suicide (MHMD-1)	• Frequent mental distress
• Adolescents with a major depressive episode in the past 12 months (MHMD-4.1)	• MHMD-2030-01 Reduce the suicide rate
Nutrition, Physical Activity, and Obesity	Obesity
• Adults meeting aerobic physical activity and muscle-strengthening objectives (PA-2.4)	
• Obesity among adults (NWS-9)	
• Obesity among children and adolescents (NWS-10.4)	• NWS-2030-03 Reduce the proportion of children and adolescents aged 2 to 19 years who have obesity
• Mean daily intake of total vegetables (NWS-15.1)	
Oral Health	Oral Health
• Children, adolescents, and adults who visited the dentist in the past year (OH-7)	• OH-2030-08 Increase the proportion of children, adolescents, and adults who use the oral health care system

continued

TABLE 4-2 Continued

HP2020 LHIs	Recommended HP2030 LHIs
Reproductive and Sexual Health	Reproductive and Sexual Health
• Sexually experienced females receiving reproductive health services (FP-7.1)	• FP-2030-07 Increase the proportion of sexually active adolescents aged 15 to 19 years who use any method of contraception at first intercourse
• Knowledge of serostatus among HIV-positive persons (HIV-13)	• HIV-2030-03 Reduce the number of new HIV diagnoses among persons of all ages
	Social Capital/Civic Engagement
	• Proportion of eligible voters who voted in the last election
	Serious Illness
	• C-2030-01 Reduce the overall cancer death rate
Social Determinants	Social Determinants
• Students graduating from high school within 4 years of starting ninth grade (AH-5.1)	• AH-2030-04 Increase the proportion of fourth grade students whose reading skills are at or above the proficient achievement level for their grade
	• SDOH-2030-03 Reduce the proportion of persons living in poverty
	• NWS-2030-01 Reduce household food insecurity
	• SDOH-2030-04 Reduce the proportion of all households that spend more than 30 percent of income on housing
Substance Abuse	Substance Abuse
• Adolescents using alcohol or illicit drugs in past 30 days (SA-13.1)	• SU-2030-03 Reduce the drug overdose death rate
• Binge drinking in past month—Adults (SA-14.3)	• SU-2030-13 Reduce the proportion of people with alcohol use disorder in the past year
Tobacco	Tobacco
• Adult cigarette smoking (TU-1.1)	• TU-2030-13 Reduce use of any tobacco products by adolescents
• Adolescent cigarette smoking in past 30 days (TU-2.2)	

NOTE: DTaP = diphtheria; Hep B = hepatitis B; Hib = haemophilus influenzae type B; MMR = measles, mumps, rubella.
SOURCE: HealthyPeople.gov, 2019.

APPLYING PHASE 2 OF THE LHI SELECTION CRITERIA TO THE PROPOSED LHI SET

The final question the committee must answer is how does the set of 34 LHIs compare to the Phase 2 criteria defined by the SAC:

- The LHIs represent a balanced portfolio or cohesive set of indicators of health and well-being across the lifespan.
- The LHIs are balanced between common, upstream root causes of poor health and well-being and measures of high-priority health states.
- The LHIs are amenable to policy, environmental, and systems interventions at the local, state, tribal, and national levels.
- The LHIs are understandable and will resonate with diverse stakeholders to drive action.

The 34 measures in the set include both measures of health and measures of well-being. For example, there are several measures of health outcomes (e.g., cancer death rate), measures of self-rated health and disability, and measures of mental distress, but there are also measures of child and adult well-being (prevalence of ACEs, the Cantril Scale). The set of LHIs includes measures that apply to different age groups, from infants and children, to older adults.

The proposed LHIs also include a combination of upstream root causes (e.g., poverty, residential segregation, educational attainment) and of high-priority health states (e.g., overdose deaths, rate of hypertension). The set of LHIs may be mapped to all categories of interventions and one or more geographic levels. The tobacco use LHI tracks the effect of tobacco policies implemented at the national and state levels (e.g., raising the minimum age for purchase to 21 years of age, implementing regulatory strategies to address youth vaping) (FDA, 2019; IOM, 2015a). The topic residential segregation has two LHIs, measures that may be tracked at the neighborhood, city, and county level (Logan and Parman, 2014). The HVI proposed to track climate change-associated health effects may be measured at the national, state, and local level, and is amenable to a variety of environmental interventions, including approaches for cooling urban heat islands (Harlan and Ruddell, 2011; Rotzer et al., 2019). Finally, a number of the LHIs may be used for international comparisons. These include life expectancy, the measures of self-rated health and well-being, and the HVI.

5

Conclusion

The committee is grateful for the opportunity to help the Department of Health and Human Services, the Federal Interagency Workgroup, and their federal, state, and local partners and stakeholders in the important *Healthy People 2030* effort. The committee hopes that its proposed set of Leading Health Indicators will be informative in the selection of the final set, which will serve as a North Star for the nation's population health improvement efforts.

References

100 Million Healthier Lives and NCVHS (National Committee on Vital and Health Statistics). 2019. *Well-Being in the Nation (WIN) measurement framework: Measures for improving health, well-being, and equity across sectors*. https://www.winmeasures.org/statistics/winmeasures (accessed June 3, 2019).

AACR (American Association for Cancer Research). 2019. How can identifying and measuring exposures to environmental carcinogens help prevent cancer? In *Cancer Research Catalyst*. American Association for Cancer Research. https://www.aacr.org/professionals/blog/how-can-identifying-and-measuring-exposures-to-environmental-carcinogens-help-prevent-cancer (accessed January 5, 2020).

Acevedo-Garcia, D. 2000. Residential segregation and the epidemiology of infectious diseases. *Social Science & Medicine* 51(8):1143–1161.

AHRQ (Agency for Healthcare Research and Quality). 2001. *AHRQ quality indicators—guide to quality prevention indicators: Hospital admission for ambulatory care sensitive conditions*. Rockville, MD: Agency for Healthcare Research and Quality. AHRQ Pub. No. 02-R0203. https://www.ahrq.gov/downloads/pub/ahrqqi/pqiguide.pdf (accessed December 14, 2019).

Anderson, G. F., P. Hussey, and V. Petrosyan. 2019. It's still the prices, stupid: Why the US spends so much on health care, and a tribute to Uwe Reinhardt. *Health Affairs (Millwood)* 38(1):87–95.

ASPE (Office of the Assistant Secretary for Planning and Evaluation). 2018. *Comparison of U.S. and international prices for top Medicare Part B drugs by total expenditures*. Washington, DC: Office of the Assistant Secretary for Planning and Evaluation, Department of Health and Human Services.

Auerbach, D. I., and A. L. Kellermann. 2011. A decade of health care cost growth has wiped out real income gains for an average US family. *Health Affairs* 30(9):1630–1636.

Baicker, K. 2001. Government decision-making and the incidence of federal mandates. *Journal of Public Economics* 82(2):147–194.

Ballard, P. J., L. T. Hoyt, and M. C. Pachucki. 2019. Impacts of adolescent and young adult civic engagement on health and socioeconomic status in adulthood. *Child Development* 90(4):1138–1154.

BARHII (Bay Area Regional Health Inequities Initiative). 2015. *Applying social determinants of health indicator data for advancing health equity: A guide for local health department epidemiologists and public health professionals.* Oakland, CA: BARHII.

Beck, A. N., B. K. Finch, S. F. Lin, R. A. Hummer, and R. K. Masters. 2014. Racial disparities in self-rated health: Trends, explanatory factors, and the changing role of socio-demographics. *Social Science & Medicine* 104:163–177. doi: 10.1016/j.socscimed.2013.11.021.

Bellis, M. A., K, Hughes, K. Ford, G. Ramos Rodriguez, D. Sethi, and J. Passmore. 2019. Life course health consequences and associated annual costs of adverse childhood experiences across Europe and North America: A systematic review and meta-analysis. *Lancet Public Health* 4(1):e517–e528.

Berry, K. N., H. A. Huskamp, H. H. Goldman, L. Rutkow, and C. L. Barry. 2017. Litigation provides clues to ongoing challenges in implementing insurance parity. *Journal of Health Politics, Policy and Law* 42(6):1065–1098.

Billings, J., G. M. Anderson, and L. S. Newman. 1996. Recent findings on preventable hospitalizations. *Health Affairs (Millwood)* 15(3):239–249.

Blakely, T. A., B. P. Kennedy, and I. Kawachi. 2001. Socioeconomic inequality in voting participation and self-rated health. *American Journal of Public Health* 91(1):99–104.

Borrescio-Higa, F. 2015. Can Walmart make us healthier? Prescription drug prices and health care utilization. *Journal of Health Economics* 44:37–53.

Braveman, P. 1998. *Monitoring inequities in health: A policy-oriented approach in low- and middle-income countries.* Geneva, Switzerland: World Health Organization.

Braveman P., E. Arkin, T. Orleans, D. Proctor, and A. Plough. 2017. What is health equity? And what difference does a definition make? Princeton, NJ: Robert Wood Johnson Foundation. https://www.rwjf.org/en/library/research/2017/05/what-is-health-equity-.html (accessed December 20, 2019).

Brown, T. T. 2016. Returns on investment in California county departments of public health. *American Journal of Public Health* 106(8):1477–1482.

Brulle, R. J., and D. N. Pellow. 2006. Environmental justice: Human health and environmental inequalities. *Annual Review of Public Health* 27:103–124.

Cantril, H. 1965. *The pattern of human concerns.* New Brunswick, NJ: Rutgers University Press.

Case, A., and A. Deaton. 2017. Mortality and morbidity in the 21st century. *Brookings Papers on Economic Activity* Spring 2017:397–476. https://www.brookings.edu/wp-content/uploads/2017/08/casetextsp17bpea.pdf (accessed November 13, 2019).

CDC (Centers for Disease Control and Prevention). 2008. Racial/ethnic disparities in self-rated health status among adults with and without disabilities—United States, 2004–2006. *Morbidity and Mortality Weekly Report* 57(39):1069–1073.

CDC. 2011. *High blood pressure and cholesterol: Out of control.* https://www.cdc.gov/vitalsigns/cardiovasculardisease/index.html (accessed January 5, 2020).

CDC. 2018. *Well-being concepts.* https://www.cdc.gov/hrqol/wellbeing.htm (accessed November 13, 2019).

CDC. 2019. *Preventing adverse childhood experiences (ACEs): Leveraging the best available evidence.* Atlanta, GA: National Center for Injury Prevention and Control.

Chetty, R., and N. Hendren. 2017. The impacts of neighborhoods on intergenerational mobility I: Childhood exposure effects. NBER Working Paper No. 23001. *The Quarterly Journal of Economics* 133(3):1107–1162.

Chetty, R., M. Stepner, S. Abraham, S. Lin, B. Scuderi, N. Turner, A. Bergeron, and D. Cutler. 2016. The association between income and life expectancy in the United States, 2001–2014. *JAMA* 315(16):1750–1766.

Chetty, R., N. Hendren, M. R. Jones, and S. R. Porter. 2019. Race and economic opportunity in the United States: An intergenerational perspective. NBER Working Paper No. 24441. https://www.nber.org/papers/w24441 (accessed December 14, 2019).

Clinton, J. D., and M. W. Sances. 2018. The politics of policy: The initial mass political effects of medicaid expansion in the states. *American Political Science Review* 112(1):167–185.

CMS (Centers for Medicare & Medicaid Services). 2015. *2014 measure information about the acute and chronic ambulatory care–sensitive condition composite measures, calculated for the value-based payment modifier program.*

CMS.gov. 2018. *National health expenditure data—historical.* https://www.cms.gov/Research-Statistics-Data-and-Systems/Statistics-Trends-and-Reports/NationalHealthExpendData/NationalHealthAccountHistorical.html (accessed November 14, 2019).

Cohen, R. A., P. Boersma, and A. Vahratian. 2019. *Strategies used by adults aged 18–64 to reduce their prescription drug costs, 2017.* National Center for Health Statistics, NCHS Data Brief 333.

County Health Rankings and Roadmaps. 2019. *2019 County Health Rankings: Key findings report.* University of Wisconsin Population Health Institute and Robert Wood Johnson Foundation.

Cullen, K. A., B. K. Ambrose, A. S. Gentzke, B. J. Apelberg, A. Jamal, and B. A. King. 2018. Notes from the field: Use of electronic cigarettes and any tobacco product among middle and high school students—United States, 2011–2018. *Morbidity and Mortality Weekly Report* 67:1276–1277.

Dai, D. 2010. Black residential segregation, disparities in spatial access to health care facilities, and late-stage breast cancer diagnosis in metropolitan Detroit. *Health & Place* 16(5):1038–1051.

Denny, K. J., and O. M. Doyle. 2007. "... Take up thy bed, and vote." Measuring the relationship between voting behaviour and indicators of health. *European Journal of Public Health* 17(4):400–401.

Desalvo, K. B., N. Bloser, K. Reynolds, J. He, and P. Muntner. 2006. Mortality prediction with a single general self-rated health question. *Journal of General Internal Medicine* 21(3):267–275.

Ebi, K. L., C. Boyer, K. J. Bowen, H. Frumkin, and J. Hess. 2018. Monitoring and evaluation indicators for climate change–related health impacts, risks, adaptation, and resilience. *International Journal of Environmental Research and Public Health* 15(9):1943.

Ehsan, M. R. 2018. What matters? Non-electoral youth political participation in austerity Britain. *Societies* 8(4):101.

EPA (Environmental Protection Agency). 2017. *Heat-related deaths.* https://www.epa.gov/sites/production/files/2017-01/documents/heat-deaths_documentation.pdf (accessed November 3, 2019).

FDA (Food and Drug Administration). 2019. *How FDA is regulating e-cigarettes.* https://www.fda.gov/news-events/fda-voices-perspectives-fda-leadership-and-experts/how-fda-regulating-e-cigarettes (accessed November 21, 2019).

Felitti, V. J., R. F. Anda, D. Nordenberg, D. F. Williamson, A. M. Spitz, V. Edwards, M. P. Koss, and J. S. Marks. 1998. Relationship of childhood abuse and household dysfunction to many of the leading causes of death in adults. The adverse childhood experiences (ACE) study. *American Journal of Preventive Medicine* 14(4):245–258.

Friedman, S., H. Xu, J. M. Harwood, F. Azocar, B. Hurley, and S. L. Ettner. 2017. The Mental Health Parity and Addiction Equity Act evaluation study: Impact on specialty behavioral healthcare utilization and spending among enrollees with substance use disorders. *Journal of Substance Abuse Treatment* 80:67–78.

Fuller-Thomson, E., A. Nuru-Jeter, M. Minkler, and J. M. Guralnik. 2009. Black-white disparities in disability among older americans: Further untangling the role of race and socioeconomic status. *Journal of Aging and Health* 21(5):677–698.

Galarraga, J. E., R. Mutter, and J. M. Pines. 2015. Costs associated with ambulatory care sensitive conditions across hospital-based settings. *Academic Emergency Medicine* 22(2):172–181.

Gallup. n.d. *Understanding how Gallup uses the Cantril scale: Development of the "thriving, struggling, suffering" categories*. https://news.gallup.com/poll/122453/understanding-gallup-uses-cantril-scale.aspx (accessed November 13, 2019).

Gee, G. C., and D. C. Payne-Sturges. 2004. Environmental health disparities: A framework integrating psychosocial and environmental concepts. *Environmental Health Perspectives* 112(17):1645–1653.

Geronimus, A. T., M. Hicken, D. Keene, and J. Bound. 2006. "Weathering" and age patterns of allostatic load scores among blacks and whites in the United States. *American Journal of Public Health* 96(5):826–833.

Goodman, M., S. Lyons, L. T. Dean, C. Arroyo, and J. A. Hipp. 2018. How segregation makes us fat: Food behaviors and food environment as mediators of the relationship between residential segregation and individual body mass index. *Frontiers in Public Health* 6:92.

Gray, C. L., D. T. Lobdell, K. M. Rappazzo, Y. Jian, J. S. Jagai, L. C. Messer, A. P. Patel, S. A. DeFlorio-Barker, C. Lyttle, J. Solway, and A. Rzhetsky. 2018a. Associations between environmental quality and adult asthma prevalence in medical claims data. *Environmental Research* 166:529–536.

Gray, C. L., L. C. Messer, K. M. Rappazzo, J. S. Jagai, S. C. Grabich, and D. T. Lobdell. 2018b. The association between physical inactivity and obesity is modified by five domains of environmental quality in U.S. adults: A cross-sectional study. *PLOS ONE* 13(8):e0203301.

Habibov, N., and R. Weaver. 2014. Endogenous social capital and self-rated health: Results from Canada's general social survey. *Health Sociology Review* 23(3):219–231.

Handler, A., M. Issel, and B. Turnock. 2001. A conceptual framework to measure performance of the public health system. *American Journal of Public Health* 91(8):1235–1239.

Harlan, S. L., and D. M. Ruddell. 2011. Climate change and health in cities: Impacts of heat and air pollution and potential co-benefits from mitigation and adaptation. *Current Opinion in Environmental Sustainability* 3(3):126–134.

Haselswerdt, J. 2017. Expanding Medicaid, expanding the electorate: The Affordable Care Act's short-term impact on political participation. *Journal of Health Politics, Policy and Law* 42(4):667–695.

Hayanga, A. J., A. K. Waljee, H. E. Kaiser, D. C. Chang, and A. M. Morris. 2009. Racial clustering and access to colorectal surgeons, gastroenterologists, and radiation oncologists by African Americans and Asian Americans in the United States: A county-level data analysis. *Archives of Surgery* 144(6):532–535.

HealthyPeople.gov. 2019. *Health-related quality of life & well-being*. https://www.healthypeople.gov/2020/topics-objectives/topic/health-related-quality-of-life-well-being (accessed November 21, 2019).

HealthyPeople.gov. n.d. *General health status*. https://www.healthypeople.gov/2020/about/foundation-health-measures/general-health-status#top (accessed November 21, 2019).

Helliwell, J., H. Huang, and S. Wang. 2019. Changing world happiness. In *World happiness report 2019*. New York: Sustainable Development Solutions Network. Pp. 10–45.

Hernandez, D. 2012. *Double jeopardy: How third grade reading skills and poverty influence high school graduation*. The Annie E. Casey Foundation.

HHS (Department of Health and Human Services). 2018. *Proposed objectives for inclusion in* Healthy People 2030.

HHS. n.d. *Search* Healthy People 2020 *evidence-based resources*. https://www.healthypeople.gov/2020/tools-resources/evidence-based-resources#ratings (accessed May 29, 2019).

Himmelstein, D. U., and S. Woolhandler. 2016. Public health's falling share of US health spending. *American Journal of Public Health* 106(1):56–57.

HUD (Department of Housing and Urban Development). 2015. *Healthy Communities Index (HCI) core indicators*.

Hughes, K., M. A. Bellis, K. A. Hardcastle, D. Sethi, A. Butchart, C. Mikton, L. Jones, and M. P. Dunne. 2017. The effect of multiple adverse childhood experiences on health: A systematic review and meta-analysis. *Lancet Public Health* 2(8):e356–e366.

Iceland, J., D. Weinberg, and E. Steinmetz. 2002. Measures of residential segregation. In *Racial and ethnic residential segregation in the United States: 1980–2000*. U.S. Census Bureau.

IOM (Institute of Medicine). 2003. *Unequal treatment: Confronting racial and ethnic disparities in health care*. Washington, DC: The National Academies Press.

IOM. 2011. *For the public's health: The role of measurement in action and accountability*. Washington, DC: The National Academies Press.

IOM. 2012. *For the public's health: Investing in a healthier future*. Washington, DC: The National Academies Press.

IOM. 2015a. *Public health implications of raising the minimum age of legal access to tobacco products*. Washington, DC: The National Academies Press.

IOM. 2015b. *Vital signs: Core metrics for health and health care progress*. Washington, DC: The National Academies Press.

Izenberg, J. M., M. S. Mujahid, and I. H. Yen. 2018. Health in changing neighborhoods: A study of the relationship between gentrification and self-rated health in the state of California. *Health & Place* 52:188–195.

Jagai, J. S., L. C. Messer, K. M. Rappazzo, C. L. Gray, S. C. Grabich, and D. T. Lobdell. 2017. County-level cumulative environmental quality associated with cancer incidence. *Cancer* 123(15):2901–2908.

Jian, Y., L. C. Messer, J. S. Jagai, K. M. Rappazzo, C. L. Gray, S. C. Grabich, and D. T. Lobdell. 2017a. Associations between environmental quality and mortality in the contiguous United States, 2000–2005. *Environmental Health Perspectives* 125(3):355–362.

Jian, Y., C. Y. H. Wu, and J. M. Gohlke. 2017b. Effect modification by environmental quality on the association between heatwaves and mortality in alabama, United States. *International Journal of Environmental Research and Public Health* 14(10):1143.

Jones, K., B. Siegel, H. Mead, L. Cartwright-Smith, C. Ramos, and K. Woods. 2008. *Racial and ethnic disparities in U.S. health care: A chartbook*. Washington, DC: The Commonwealth Fund.

Kaplan, R. M., V. J. Howard, J. J. Manly, and G. Howard. 2017. Comparison of simple efficient clinical and self-reported predictors of mortality in a national United States cohort. *Journal of Epidemiological Research* 3(2):23.

Kershaw, K. N., W. R. Robinson, P. Gordon-Larsen, M. T. Hicken, D. C. Goff, M. R. Carnethon, C. I. Kiefe, S. Sidney, and A. V. Diez Roux. 2017. Association of changes in neighborhood-level racial residential segregation with changes in blood pressure among black adults: The CARDIA study. *JAMA Internal Medicine* 177(7):996–1002.

Klar, M., and T. Kasser. 2009. Some benefits of being an activist: Measuring activism and its role in psychological well-being. *Political Psychology* 30(5):755–777.

Kramer, M., and C. Hogue. 2009. Is segregation bad for your health? *Epidemiologic Reviews* 31:178–194.

Landrine, H., I. Corral, J. G. L. Lee, J. T. Efird, M. B. Hall, and J. J. Bess. 2017. Residential segregation and racial cancer disparities: A systematic review. *Journal of Racial and Ethnic Health Disparities* 4(6):1195–1205.

Lansford, J. E., K. A. Dodge, G. S. Pettit, and J. E. Bates. 2016. A public health perspective on school dropout and adult outcomes: A prospective study of risk and protective factors from age 5 to 27 years. *Journal of Adolescent Health* 58(6):652–658.

LaVeist, T. A., D. Gaskin, and P. Richard. 2011. Estimating the economic burden of racial health inequalities in the United States. *International Journal of Health Services* 41(2):231–238.

Leider, J. P., N. Alfonso, B. Resnick, E. Brady, J. M. McCullough, and D. Bishai. 2018. Assessing the value of 40 years of local public expenditures on health. *Health Affairs (Millwood)* 37(4):560–569.

Lobdell, D. T., J. S. Jagai, K. Rappazzo, and L. C. Messer. 2011. Data sources for an environmental quality index: Availability, quality, and utility. *American Journal of Public Health* 101(Suppl 1):S277–S285.

Lobdell, D., J. Jagai, L. Messer, K. Rappazzo, K. Messier, G. Smith, S. Pierson, B. Rosenbaum, and M. Murphy. 2014. *Environmental Quality Index—overview report.* Washington, DC: Environmental Protection Agency. EPA/600/R-14/305.

Lobdell, D., Y. Jian, C. Gray, S. Grabich, J. Jagai, K. Rappazzo, and L. Messer. 2016. Racial/ethnic disparities in the associations between environmental quality and mortality in the contiguous U.S. *International Society for Environmental Epidemiology Conference Abstracts* No. P1-271.

Logan, T. D., and J. M. Parman 2014. Measuring residential segregation. Yale University white paper. https://economics.yale.edu/sites/default/files/segregation-measures_03-24-14.pdf (accessed January 5, 2020).

Madrigano, J., K. Ito, S. Johnson, P. L. Kinney, and T. Matte. 2015. A case-only study of vulnerability to heat wave-related mortality in New York City (2000–2011). *Environmental Health Perspectives* 123(7):672–678. doi: 10.1289/ehp.1408178.

Martin, A. B., M. Hartman, B. Washington, and A. Catlin. 2019. National health care spending in 2017: Growth slows to post-great recession rates; share of GDO stabilizes. *Health Affairs (Millwood)* 38(1):101377hlthaff201805085.

Massey, D., and N. Denton. 1993. *American apartheid: Segregation and the making of the underclass.* Cambridge, MA: Harvard University Press.

Masters, R., E. Anwar, B. Collins, R. Cookson, and S. Capewell. 2017. Return on investment of public health interventions: A systematic review. *Journal of Epidemiology and Community Health* 71(8):827–834.

Mays, G. P., and C. B. Mamaril. 2017. Public health spending and Medicare resource use: A longitudinal analysis of U.S. communities. *Health Services Research* 52(Suppl 2):2357–2377.

Mays, G. P., and S. A. Smith. 2011. Evidence links increases in public health spending to declines in preventable deaths. *Health Affairs* 30(8):1585–1593.

Mays, V. M., S. D. Cochran, and N. W. Barnes. 2007. Race, race-based discrimination, and health outcomes among African Americans. *Annual Review of Psychology* 58:201–225.

McCullough, J. M. 2019. Declines in spending despite positive returns on investment: Understanding public health's wrong pocket problem. *Frontiers in Public Health* 7:159.

Measure of America. 2018. Methodological note. In *Measuring America: 10 Years and Counting.*

Mehra, R., L. M. Boyd, and J. R. Ickovics. 2017. Racial residential segregation and adverse birth outcomes: A systematic review and meta-analysis. *Social Science & Medicine* 191:237–250.

Merrick, M. T., D. C. Ford, K. A. Ports, A. S. Guinn, J. Chen, J. Klevens, M. Metzler, C. M. Jones, T. R. Simon, V. M. Daniel, P. Ottley, and J. A. Mercy. 2019. Vital signs: Estimated proportion of adult health problems attributable to adverse childhood experiences and implications for prevention—25 states, 2015–2017. *Morbidity and Mortality Weekly Report* 68(44):999–1005.

Mersky, J. P., and C. E. Janczewski. 2018. Racial and ethnic differences in the prevalence of adverse childhood experiences: Findings from a low-income sample of U.S. women. *Child Abuse & Neglect* 76:480–487.

Messer, L. C., J. S. Jagai, K. M. Rappazzo, and D. T. Lobdell. 2014. Construction of an environmental quality index for public health research. *Environmental Health* 13(1):39.

Meyer, A. M., M. Davis, and G. P. Mays. 2012. Defining organizational capacity for public health services and systems research. *Journal of Public Health Management & Practice* 18(6):535–544.

Morello-Frosch, R., and B. M. Jesdale. 2006. Separate and unequal: Residential segregation and estimated cancer risks associated with ambient air toxics in U.S. metropolitan areas. *Environmental Health Perspectives* 114(3):386–393. doi: 10.1289/ehp.8500.

Murayama, H., Y. Fujiwara, and I. Kawachi. 2012. Social capital and health: A review of prospective multilevel studies. *Journal of Epidemiology* 22(3):179–187.

NASEM (National Academies of Sciences, Engineering, and Medicine). 2017. *Communities in action: Pathways to health equity*. Washington, DC: The National Academies Press.

NASEM. 2019a. *A roadmap to reducing child poverty*. Washington, DC: The National Academies Press.

NASEM. 2019b. *Vibrant and healthy kids: Aligning science, practice, and policy to advance health equity*. Washington, DC: The National Academies Press.

NASEM. 2019c. *Criteria for selecting the Leading Health Indicators for* Healthy People 2030. Washington, DC: The National Academies Press.

NCTSN (The National Child Traumatic Stress Network). n.d. *Home page*. https://www.nctsn.org (accessed November 21, 2019).

NIMHD (National Institute on Minority Health and Health Disparities). 2017. *NIMHD research framework*. https://nimhd.nih.gov/about/overview/research-framework/nimhd-framework.html (accessed January 13, 2020).

Nobles, C. J., S. E. Valentine, E. D. Zepeda, Y. Wang, E. M. Ahles, D. L. Shtasel and L. Marques. 2017. Residential segregation and mental health among Latinos in a nationally representative survey. *Journal of Epidemiology and Community Health* 71(4):318–323.

NORC. 2019. Healthy People 2030 *public comment analysis*. Chicago, IL: University of Chicago.

NRC (National Research Council). 2014. *Civic engagement and social cohesion measuring dimensions of social capital to inform policy*. Washington, DC: The National Academies Press.

NRC and IOM (Institute of Medicine). 2013. *U.S. health in international perspective: Shorter lives, poorer health*. Washington, DC: The National Academies Press.

ODPHP (Office of Disease Prevention and Health Promotion). 2019. Secretary's advisory committee on national health promotion and disease prevention objectives for 2030. Meeting slides, June 26, 2019. https://www.healthypeople.gov/sites/default/files/508%20Compliant%20Slides%20for%20June%202019%20Committee%20Meeting.pdf (accessed November 13, 2019).

OECD (Organisation for Economic Co-operation and Development). 2011. *OECD launches new report on measuring well-being*. https://www.oecd.org/newsroom/oecdlaunchesnewreportonmeasuringwell-being.htm (accessed November 13, 2019).

OECD. 2013. *OECD guidelines on measuring subjective well-being*. Paris, France: OECD Publishing.

OECD. 2017a. *Better life index 2017 definitions and metadata*. https://www.oecd.org/statistics/OECD-Better-Life-Index-2017-definitions.pdf (accessed 2019).

OECD. 2017b. *Health at a glance 2017: Oecd indicators*. Paris, France: OECD Publishing.

O'Neil, S. S., T. Lake, A. Merrill, A. Wilson, D. A. Mann, and L. M. Bartnyska. 2010. Racial disparities in hospitalizations for ambulatory care–sensitive conditions. *American Journal of Preventive Medicine* 38(4):381–388.

Orszag, P., and T. Kane. 2003. *Higher education spending: The role of Medicaid and the business cycle*. Washington, DC: The Brookings Institution.

Pickett, K. E., and M. Pearl. 2001. Multilevel analyses of neighbourhood socioeconomic context and health outcomes: A critical review. *Journal of Epidemiology and Community Health* 55(2):111–122.

PolicyLink and USC PERE (University of California Program for Environmental and Regional Equity). 2018. The National Equity Atlas.

Prevention Institute. 2015. *Measuring what works to achieve health equity: Metrics for the determinants of health.*

Rappazzo, K. M., L. C. Messer, J. S. Jagai, C. L. Gray, S. C. Grabich, and D. T. Lobdell. 2015. The associations between environmental quality and preterm birth in the United States, 2000–2005: A cross-sectional analysis. *Environmental Health: A Global Access Science Source* 14:50.

Reichel, C. 2018. How health affects voter turnout: A research roundup. In *Journalist's Resource: Research on Today's News.* Harvard Kennedy School, Shorenstein Center on Media, Politics and Public Policy.

Riley, W. J., E. M. Lownik, F. D. Scutchfield, G. P. Mays, L. C. Corso, and L. M. Beitsch. 2012. Public health department accreditation: Setting the research agenda. *American Journal of Preventive Medicine* 2(3):263–271.

Rotzer, T., M. A. Rahman, A. Moser-Reischl, S. Pauleit, and H. Pretzsch. 2019. Process based simulation of tree growth and ecosystem services of urban trees under present and future climate conditions. *Science of the Total Environment* 676:651–664.

SAC (Secretary's Advisory Committee on National Health Promotion and Disease Prevention Objectives for 2030). 2010. *Evidence-based clinical and public health: Generating and applying the evidence.* https://www.healthypeople.gov/sites/default/files/EvidenceBasedClinicalPH2010.pdf (accessed May 29, 2019).

SAC. 2018a. *Objective selection criteria.* https://www.healthypeople.gov/sites/default/files/ObjectiveSelectionCriteria508_1.17.19.pdf (accessed May 17, 2019).

SAC. 2018b. *Issue briefs to inform development and implementation of* Healthy People 2030. https://www.healthypeople.gov/sites/default/files/HP2030_Committee-Combined-Issue%20Briefs_2019-508c_0.pdf (accessed April 24, 2019).

SAC. 2019. *Report #7: Assessment and recommendations for proposed objectives for* Healthy People 2030.

Sampson, R. J., J. D. Morenoff, and T. Gannon-Rowley. 2002. Assessing "neighborhood effects": Social processes and new directions in research. *Annual Review of Sociology* 28(1):443–478.

Schenck, A. P., A. M. Meyer, T.-M. Kuo, and D. Cilenti. 2015. Building the evidence for decision-making: The relationship between local public health capacity and community mortality. *American Journal of Public Health* 105(S2):S211–S216.

Scutchfield, F. D., M. W. Bhandari, N. A. Lawhorn, C. D. Lamberth, and R. C. Ingram. 2009. Public health performance. *American Journal of Preventive Medicine* 36(3):266–272.

Sensenig, A. L. 2007. Refining estimates of public health spending as measured in national health expenditures accounts: The United States experience. *Journal of Public Health Management & Practice* 13(2):103–114.

Shah, S. N., E. T. Russo, T. R. Earl, and T. Kuo. 2014. Measuring and monitoring progress toward health equity: Local challenges for public health. *Preventing Chronic Disease* 11:E159.

Singh, S. 2014. Public health spending and population health. *American Journal of Public Health* 47(5):634–640.

Singh-Manoux, A., N. E. Adler, and M. G. Marmot. 2003. Subjective social status: Its determinants and its association with measures of ill-health in the Whitehall II study. *Social Science & Medicine* 56(6):1321–1333.

Singh-Manoux, A., M. G. Marmot, and N. E. Adler. 2005. Does subjective social status predict health and change in health status better than objective status? *Psychosomatic Medicine* 67(6):855–861.

Stranges, E., and C. Stocks. 2008. *Potentially preventable hospitalizations for acute and chronic conditions.* Rockville, MD: Agency for Healthcare Research and Quality.

TFAH (Trust for America's Health). 2006. *Shortchanging America's health 2006: A state-by-state look at how federal public health dollars are spent.*

The Annie E. Casey Foundation. 2013. *Early reading research confirmed: A research update on the importance of third-grade reading.* https://www.aecf.org/resources/early-warning-confirmed (accessed November 25, 2019).

The Annie E. Casey Foundation. 2019. *Kids count data book 2019: State trends in child well-being.*

Tikkanen, R. *Multinational comparisons of health systems data, 2017.* The Commonwealth Fund. https://www.commonwealthfund.org/publications/other-publication/2017/nov/multinational-comparisons-health-systems-data-2017 (accessed December 20, 2019).

UNDP: Human Development Reports. n.d. *Human development data (1990–2018)* http://hdr.undp.org/en/data (accessed November 11, 2019).

van der Vorst, A., G. A. Zijlstra, N. Witte, D. Duppen, A. E. Stuck, G. I. Kempen, and J. M. Schols. 2016. Limitations in activities of daily living in community-dwelling people aged 75 and over: A systematic literature review of risk and protective factors. *PLOS ONE* 11(10):e0165127.

Verma, R., S. Clark, J. Leider, and D. Bishai. 2017. Impact of state public health spending on disease incidence in the United States from 1980 to 2009. *Health Services Research* 52(1):176–190.

Watts, N., M. Amann, N. Arnell, et al. 2019. The 2019 report of The Lancet Countdown on health and climate change: ensuring that the health of a child born today is not defined by a changing climate. *Lancet* 394(10211):1836–1878.

Weinberg, D., J. Iceland, and E. Steinmetz. 2002. Measurement of segregation by the US Bureau of the Census. In *Racial and ethnic residential segregation in the United States: 1980–2000.* U.S. Census Bureau. https://www.census.gov/hhes/www/housing/housing_patterns/pdf/massey.pdf (accessed November 22, 2019).

Wen, H., K. J. Johnston, L. Allen, and T. M. Waters. 2019. Medicaid expansion associated with reductions in preventable hospitalizations. *Health Affairs (Millwood)* 38(11):1845–1849.

WHO (World Health Organization). 2010. *A conceptual framework for action on the social determinants of health.* https://www.who.int/social_determinants/publications/9789241500852/en (accessed October 25, 2019).

WHO. 2012. *Measurement of and target-setting for well-being: An initiative by the WHO regional office for Europe: Second meeting of the expert group.* Paris, France, June 25–26, 2012.

WHO. 2017. *Cardiovascular diseases (CVDs).* https://www.who.int/news-room/fact-sheets/detail/cardiovascular-diseases-(cvds) (accessed January 5, 2020).

Wilkinson, R., and M. Marmot. 2003. *Social determinants of health: The solid facts.* Geneva, Switzerland: World Health Organization.

Williams, D. R., and C. Collins. 2001. Racial residential segregation: A fundamental cause of racial disparities in health. *Public Health Reports* 116(5):404–416.

Wisconsin DHS (Department of Health Services). 2017. *Vulnerability indexes.* https://www.dhs.wisconsin.gov/climate/wihvi.htm (accessed December 12, 2019).

Wong Croal, N., B. Smedley, D. Andrulis, D., S. Woolf, N. Siddiqui, K. Wilson, M. Turner, and A. Stelter. 2018. *The HOPE Initiative: Brief Report.* https://www.nationalcollaborative.org/wp-content/uploads/2018/07/hope_brief_report_final.pdf (accessed June 5, 2019).

Woolf, S., D. Chapman, L. Hill, H. Schoomaker, D. Wheeler, L. Snellings, and J. Hyung Lee. 2018. *Uneven opportunities: How conditions for wellness vary across the metropolitan Washington region.* Virginia Commonwealth University.

Woolf, S. H., R. E. Johnson, R. L. Phillips, and M. Philipsen. 2007. Giving everyone the health of the educated: An examination of whether social change would save more lives than medical advances. *American Journal of Public Health* 97(4):679–683.

Appendix A

Committee Member Biosketches[1]

GEORGE J. ISHAM, M.D., M.S. (*Chair*), is currently a Senior Fellow at the HealthPartners Institute in Minneapolis, Minnesota. His areas of interest include understanding how health is created in populations and how to improve health and health care quality and financing. He is formerly a Senior Advisor (2012–2017) and Medical Director and Chief Health Officer (1993–2012) at HealthPartners. He is also currently a Senior Advisor to the Alliance of Community Health Plans and a member of the advisory board for the Center for Health Economics and Policy at FTI Consulting. Dr. Isham is an elected member of the National Academy of Medicine and was designated as a National Associate of the Institute of Medicine in 2003 in recognition of his contribution to its work. He has chaired the National Academies' Roundtable on Population Health Improvement and the Roundtable on Health Literacy; chaired, served, and been a reviewer for a number of consensus committee reports; and participated in a number of National Academies workshops. Dr. Isham has been active in health policy, serving as a former member of the Centers for Disease Control and Prevention's (CDC's) Task Force on Community Preventive Services, as a member of the Agency for Healthcare Research and Quality's U.S. Preventive Services Task Force, and as a founding co-chair of the National Committee for Quality Assurance's committee on performance measurement as well as a founding co-chair of the National Quality Forum's Measurement Application Partnership. He is a founding member

[1] The members of the committee serve on the committee as individuals rather than as representatives of their respective organizations.

of the advisory board for the National Guideline Clearinghouse and has served on the Advisory Committee to the Director of CDC.

Dr. Isham earned his Bachelor of Arts in zoology and Master of Science in preventive medicine/administrative medicine from the University of Wisconsin–Madison, and his Doctor of Medicine from the University of Illinois in Chicago. He completed his internship and residency in internal medicine at the University of Wisconsin Hospital and Clinics in Madison, Wisconsin. Dr. Isham has clinical experience as a General Medical Officer in the U.S. Navy, in the general practice of internal medicine at the Freeport Clinic in Freeport, Illinois, and as a Clinical Assistant Professor of Medicine at the University of Wisconsin Hospitals and Clinics in Madison, Wisconsin.

L. EBONY BOULWARE, M.D., M.P.H., is a Professor of Medicine, Chief of the Division of General Internal Medicine in the Department of Medicine, Vice Dean for Translational Science, and Associate Vice Chancellor for Translational Research in the School of Medicine at Duke University. She received an A.B. from Vassar College, an M.D. from Duke University, and an M.P.H. from the Johns Hopkins Bloomberg School of Public Health. Dr. Boulware is a general internist and a clinical epidemiologist. She attended medical school at Duke University, completed medical training as a resident and chief resident at the University of Maryland, and completed a research fellowship at the Johns Hopkins University School of Medicine. She became a faculty member in the Johns Hopkins School of Medicine and Bloomberg School of Public Health in 2002, where she achieved the academic rank of Full Professor. In 2013, she was appointed Chief of the Division of General Internal Medicine in the Department of Medicine at Duke University. In 2015, she was appointed the inaugural Director of the Duke Clinical and Translational Science Institute, and she is the contact Principal Investigator for the Duke Clinical and Translational Science Award for Duke University. Dr. Boulware has devoted her scholarly career to studying mechanisms to improve the quality and equity of health care and health outcomes for patients and populations with chronic diseases, such as chronic kidney disease and hypertension. As part of her work, she investigates the influence of attitudinal, social, and environmental contexts on health and health outcomes. She has maintained an active research portfolio throughout her career, funded by the National Institutes of Health, the Patient-Centered Outcomes Research Institute, the Health Resources and Services Administration, the Agency for Healthcare Research and Quality, and several foundations. She has published more than 120 manuscripts, and she has mentored numerous students, fellows, and faculty members in clinical research. Dr. Boulware frequently engages community members, patients, their family members, and other stakeholders to develop and implement relevant and sustainable interventions to improve health.

GILBERT GEE, Ph.D., is a Professor in the Department of Community Health Sciences at the Fielding School of Public Health at the University of California, Los Angeles. He received his bachelor's degree in neuroscience from Oberlin College, his doctorate in health policy and management from the Johns Hopkins University, and postdoctoral training in sociology from Indiana University. His research focuses on the social determinants of health inequities of racial, ethnic, and immigrant minority populations using a multilevel and life course perspective. A primary line of his research focuses on conceptualizing and measuring racism discrimination, and in understanding how discrimination may be related to illness. He has also published more broadly on the topics of stress, neighborhoods, environmental exposures, occupational health, and Asian American populations. Current projects include the study of discrimination; racial identity and obesity among emigrants from the Philippines; the relationship between student loans and illness; and toxic exposures among Asian American participants in the National Health and Nutrition Examination Survey. His research has been honored with a group Merit Award from the National Institutes of Health for the development of multicultural measures of discrimination for health surveys. In addition, he received two Scientific and Technical Achievement Awards from the Environmental Protection Agency for development of the Stress-Exposure-Disease Framework.

MARTHE R. GOLD, M.D., M.P.H., is a Senior Scholar at The New York Academy of Medicine and the Logan Professor Emeritus in the Department of Community Health and Social Medicine at the City University of New York Medical School. A graduate of the Tufts University School of Medicine and the Columbia School of Public Health, her clinical training is in family medicine. Dr. Gold has been a primary care provider in urban and rural underserved settings. She served as Senior Policy Adviser in the Office of the Assistant Secretary for Health in the Department of Health and Human Services from 1990 to 1996, where her focus was on financing of clinical preventive services, the economics and outcomes of public health programs, and health care reform. She directed the work of the Panel on Cost-Effectiveness in Health and Medicine, an expert panel whose report remains an influential guide to cost-effectiveness methodology for academic and policy uses. Her current work focuses on patient, public, and decision maker views on using economic and comparative effectiveness information to inform health policy. A member of the National Academy of Medicine, Dr. Gold served as chair of its

Committee on Public Health Strategies to Improve Health (reports published 2010–2012) and has been a member of the Roundtable on Population Health Improvement since its inception.

SHERI JOHNSON, Ph.D. is the Director of the Population Health Institute (PHI) at the University of Wisconsin–Madison, Visiting Associate Professor, and Acting Director, County Health Rankings & Roadmaps, and the Robert Wood Johnson Foundation Culture of Health Prize. For more than 25 years Dr. Johnson has dedicated her career to partnering with children, families, community organizations, and systems to advance health and well-being. Awed by the resilience of individuals and communities, she is motivated to remove unfair obstacles and conditions that create and perpetuate health inequities. Dr. Johnson completed undergraduate studies at Brown University, earned an M.A. and a Ph.D. in clinical psychology at Boston University, and served as a Clinical Fellow in Psychology at the Harvard Medical School. She was previously the Director of Behavioral Health at Milwaukee Health Services, Inc., a federally qualified health center, and served as the Administrator and State Health Officer for the Wisconsin Division of Public Health. Immediately prior to joining the PHI, she was an Associate Professor of Pediatrics at the Medical College of Wisconsin Center for Advancement of Underserved Children, where she collaborated with diverse stakeholders to address a broad range of real-world problems.

PAULA LANTZ, Ph.D., is the Associate Dean for academic affairs and a Professor of public policy at the Ford School. She also holds an appointment as a Professor of health management and policy in the School of Public Health. Dr. Lantz, a social demographer, studies the role of public policy in improving population health. She currently directs the University of Michigan Policies for Action Research Hub, funded by the Robert Wood Johnson Foundation, which is engaged in a number of research projects investigating public policy approaches to reducing social inequities in health. Dr. Lantz is leading a project regarding the potential for and challenges associated with using social impact bonds to fund public–private partnerships aimed at improving population health. An elected member of the National Academy of Social Insurance and the National Academy of Medicine, Dr. Lantz received an M.A. in sociology from Washington University in St. Louis and an M.S. in epidemiology and a Ph.D. in sociology from the University of Wisconsin.

DARCY PHELAN-EMRICK, Dr.P.H., M.H.S., has served as the Chief Epidemiologist at the Baltimore City Health Department since 2015. She leads the Health Department's efforts to develop and track public health objectives and goals. Dr. Phelan-Emrick has been a full-time faculty member in the Department of Epidemiology at the Johns Hopkins Bloomberg School of Public Health since 2009, and she holds a joint appointment in the Department of Health, Behavior and Society. She has held prior positions in the New York City Department of Health and Mental Hygiene, The New York Academy of Medicine, and The Rockefeller University. Dr. Phelan-Emrick received her Dr.P.H. in 2009 and M.H.S. in 2005, both in epidemiology, from the Johns Hopkins Bloomberg School of Public Health.

JONATHAN S. SKINNER, Ph.D., is a health economist with experience leading several research projects funded by the National Institute on Aging. These are large-scale interdisciplinary collaborations at Dartmouth and involving partner institutions, drawing on Dartmouth's comprehensive Medicare and Medicaid datasets. Dr. Skinner's ongoing research focuses on studying the contribution of "high-tech" health care to cost growth, the diffusion of various types of medical innovations (beneficial and less so), how provider networks affect technology diffusion, and measuring efficiency in health care. A member of the National Academy of Medicine, Dr. Skinner is also a research associate and director of the Aging Program at the National Bureau of Economic Research. He has taught in Dartmouth's Department of Economics since 1995, where he serves as the James O. Freedman Presidential Professor.

Appendix B

Public Information-Gathering Meeting Agendas

MEETING ONE

Wednesday, February 27, 2019
Zoom Conferencing

2:00 pm ET **Welcome and Introductions**
George Isham, HealthPartners Institute (Committee Chair)

2:10 pm **Giving of the Charge and Context**
Carter Blakey, Office of Disease Prevention and Health Promotion, Office of the Assistant Secretary for Health, Department of Health and Human Services

2:45 pm **Q&A**

3:00 pm **Adjourn**

MEETING TWO

Friday, April 19, 2019
Zoom Conferencing

12:00 pm ET **Welcome and Introductions**
George Isham, HealthPartners Institute (Committee Chair)

12:10 pm **Update About the *Healthy People 2030* Initiative**
Don Wright, Deputy Assistant Secretary for Health, Director, Office of Disease Prevention and Health Promotion, Department of Health and Human Services (HHS)

12:20 pm **Remarks About the Work of the Secretary's Advisory Committee on National Health Promotion and Disease Prevention Objectives for 2030**
Dushanka Kleinman, Professor and Principal Associate Dean for Research, University of Maryland School of Public Health, University of Maryland (HHS Secretary's Advisory Committee[1] Co-Chair)

Nico Pronk, President, HealthPartners Institute (HHS Secretary's Advisory Committee Co-Chair)

12:50 pm **Questions from the National Academies Committee**

1:20 pm **Break**

1:35 pm **Remarks About the Work of the Subcommittee on Leading Health Indicators**
Therese Richmond, Andrea B. Laporte Professor of Nursing; Associate Dean for Research & Innovation, School of Nursing, University of Pennsylvania (Chair, Subcommittee on Leading Health Indicators)

2:05 pm **Questions from the National Academies Committee**

---

[1] Secretary's Advisory Committee on National Health Promotion and Disease Prevention Objectives for 2030.

2:35 pm **Public Comment (time permitting)**

3:00 pm **Adjourn**

MEETING THREE

May 28, 2019
Keck Center
500 Fifth Street, NW
Washington, DC 20001

9:00 am ET **Welcome and Introductions**
George Isham, HealthPartners Institute (Committee Chair)

9:15 am **Presentation from the Assistant Secretary of Health**
Don Wright, Deputy Assistant Secretary for Health, Director, Office of Disease Prevention and Health Promotion, Department of Health and Human Services (HHS)

9:30 am **Perspectives on the Purpose and Use of Leading Health Indicators (or a Small High-Level Set of Indicators for the Nation More Broadly) with Both National and Community Needs in Mind**
Moderator: Terry Richmond, University of Pennsylvania
Anita Chandra, RAND
Bobby Milstein, ReThink Health
Soma Stout, Institute for Healthcare Improvement and 100 Million Healthier Lives
Carley Riley, Cincinnati Children's and 100 Million Healthier Lives

10:30 am **Break**

10:45 am **Q&A**
Moderator: George Isham

11:10 am **Data Sources for Objectives and the Leading Health Indicators**
Moderator: Ed Sondik, formerly National Center for Health Statistics
Ali Mokdad, Institute for Health Metrics and Evaluation
Amy O'Hara, Massive Data Institute, McCourt School of Public Policy, Georgetown University

11:55 am **Q&A**
Moderator: George Isham

12:15 pm **Lunch Break**

1:15 pm **Harmonizing with Other National Metrics Sets**
Moderator: Dushanka Kleinman, University of Maryland
Tom Eckstein, Arundel Metrics
Kristen Lewis, Social Science Research Council
Marjory Givens, University of Wisconsin–Madison (via Zoom)

2:15 pm **Q&A**
Moderator: George Isham

2:40 pm **Break**

2:55 pm **Measuring Health Equity: Insights for the Leading Health Indicators**
Moderator: Nico Pronk, HealthPartners Institute
Brian Smedley, National Collaborative for Health Equity
Steve Woolf, Virginia Commonwealth University (absent)
Sarah Treuhaft, Policy Link (via Zoom)

3:40 pm **Q&A**
Moderator: George Isham

4:00 pm **Public Comment (time permitting)**

4:15 pm **Adjourn**

Appendix C

Two Social Determinants of Health Frameworks

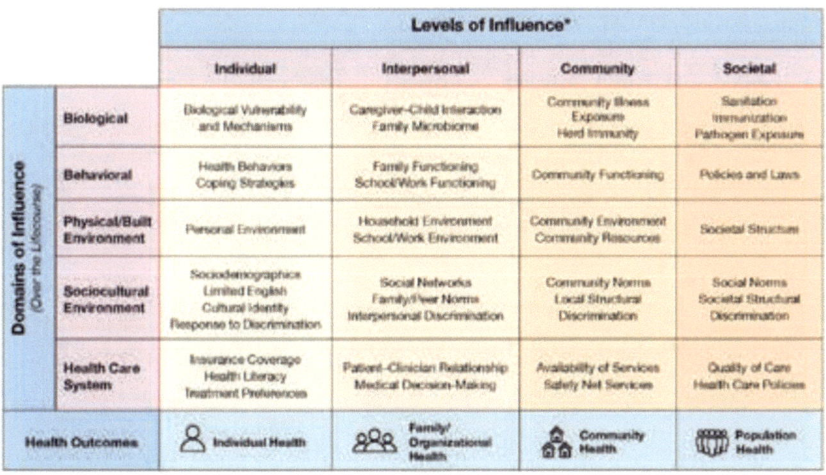

FIGURE C-1, Part 1 National Institute on Minority Health and Health Disparities research framework.
SOURCES: NIMHD, 2017; https://nimhd.nih.gov/about/overview/research-framework/nimhd-framework.html (accessed January 13, 2020).

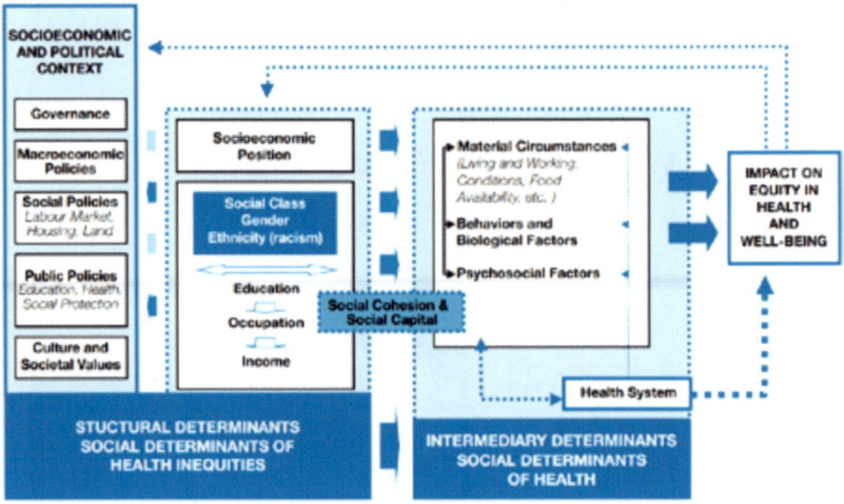

FIGURE C-1, Part 2 World Health Organization Commission on Social Determinants of Health conceptual framework.
SOURCES: WHO, 2010; https://www.who.int/sdhconference/resources/ConceptualframeworkforactiononSDH_eng.pdf (accessed July 18, 2019).

Appendix D

Leading Health Indicator Contender Form

Form used to collect Leading Health Indicator contenders from committee members.

Number	LHI Contender	Source (from Grid) (list all that apply)	Meets HP 2030 Objective Criteria (Y/N)	Meets LHI Criteria (Y/N)	Category (Report 1)	
					Life stages Health states Systems Social, physical, economic determinants	
1						
2						
3						
4						
5						
6						
7						
8						
9						
10						
11						
12						
13						
14						
15						

	Theme 1 - Cultivating Healthier Environments	Theme 2 - Increasing Knowledge and Action	Theme 3 - Closing Gaps	Theme 4 - Health and Well-Being Across the Lifespan	Comments (if any)
	Sub-level concept- note which category				
	Physical, social, economic	Shared responsibility across sectors, public health successes, evidence-based laws, policies and practices, objectives and data	Disparity, equity, health literacy	Physical, mental and social dimension, access public health, quality of public health, access to health care, quality health care	
					* See source, etc.

Appendix E

Department of Health and Human Services Proposed Objectives for Inclusion in *Healthy People 2030*

Contents

1. AH (Adolescent Health)

10 Core Objectives; 1 Developmental Objective; 7 Research Objectives

Core Objectives

Objective Number	Objective Statement	Data Source
AH-2030-01	Increase the proportion of adolescents aged 12 to 17 who received a preventive health care visit in the past 12 months	National Survey of Children's Health (NSCH), HRSA/MCHB
AH-2030-02	Increase the proportion of adolescents who have an adult in their lives with whom they can talk about serious problems	National Survey on Drug Use and Health (NSDUH), SAMHSA
AH-2030-03	Increase the proportion of students who graduate with a regular diploma 4 years after starting 9th grade	Common Core of Data (CCD), ED/NCES
AH-2030-04	Increase the proportion of 4th grade students whose reading skills are at or above the proficient achievement level for their grade	National Assessment of Educational Progress (NAEP), ED/NCES
AH-2030-05	Increase the proportion of 4th grade students whose mathematics skills are at or above the proficient achievement level for their grade	National Assessment of Educational Progress (NAEP), ED/NCES
AH-2030-06	Reduce chronic school absence among early adolescents	National Assessment of Educational Progress (NAEP), ED/NCES
AH-2030-07	Increase the proportion of students participating in the School Breakfast Program	Food Programs Reporting System (FPRS), USDA/FNS
AH-2030-08	Reduce the rate of minor and young adult perpetration of violent crimes	Uniform Crime Reporting Program (UCR), DOJ/FBI
AH-2030-09	Reduce the percentage of youth and young adults aged 16 to 24 who are neither enrolled in school nor working	Current Population Survey (CPS), Census and DOL/BLS
AH-2030-10	Increase the proportion of adolescents, ages 12-17, who spoke privately with a physician or other health care provider during their preventive medical visit in the past 12 months	National Survey of Children's Health (NSCH), HRSA/MCHB

Developmental Objectives

Objective Number	Objective Statement
AH-2030-D01	Reduce the proportion of public schools with a serious violent incident

Research Objectives

Objective Number	Objective Statement
AH-2030-R01	Increase the proportion of adolescents in foster care who exhibit positive early indicators of readiness for transition to adulthood
AH-2030-R02	Increase the proportion of students who are served under the Individuals with Disabilities Education Act who graduate high school with a diploma
AH-2030-R03	Increase the proportion ofh grade students whose reading skills are at or above the proficient achievement level for their grade
AH-2030-R04	Increase the proportion of 8th grade students whose mathematics skills are at or above the proficient achievement level for their grade
AH-2030-R05	Reduce the rate of adolescent and young adult victimization from crimes of violence
AH-2030-R06	Increase the proportion of youth with special health care needs, ages 12-17, who receive services to support their transition to adult health care
AH-2030-R07	Increase proportion of secondary schools with a start time of 8:30 AM or later

2. AHS (Access to Health Services)

9 Core Objectives; 0 Developmental Objectives; 2 Research Objectives

Core Objectives

Objective Number	Objective Statement	Data Source
AHS-2030-01	Increase the proportion of persons with medical insurance	National Health Interview Survey (NHIS), CDC/NCHS
AHS-2030-02	Increase the proportion of persons with dental insurance	National Health Interview Survey (NHIS), CDC/NCHS
AHS-2030-03	Increase the proportion of persons with prescription drug insurance	National Health Interview Survey (NHIS), CDC/NCHS
AHS-2030-04	Increase the proportion of persons with a usual primary care provider	Medical Expenditure Panel Survey (MEPS), AHRQ
AHS-2030-05	Reduce the proportion of persons who are unable to obtain or delay in obtaining necessary medical care	Medical Expenditure Panel Survey (MEPS), AHRQ
AHS-2030-06	Reduce the proportion of persons who are unable to obtain or delay in obtaining necessary dental care	Medical Expenditure Panel Survey (MEPS), AHRQ
AHS-2030-07	Reduce the proportion of persons who are unable to obtain or delay in obtaining necessary prescription medicines	Medical Expenditure Panel Survey (MEPS), AHRQ
AHS-2030-08	Increase the proportion of adults who receive appropriate evidence-based clinical preventive services	Medical Expenditure Panel Survey (MEPS)-Preventive Services Self-Administered Questionnaire,
AHS-2030-09	Reduce the proportion of all hospital emergency department visits in which the wait time to see an emergency department clinician exceeds the recommended timeframe	National Hospital Ambulatory Medical Care Survey (NHAMCS), CDC/NCHS

Research Objectives

Objective Number	Objective Statement
AHS-2030-R01	Increase the capacity of the primary care and behavioral health workforce to deliver high quality, timely, and accessible patient-centered care
AHS-2030-R02	Increase the use of telehealth to improve access to health services

3. AOCBC (Arthritis, Osteoporosis, and Chronic Back Conditions)

7 Core Objectives; 2 Developmental Objective; 0 Research Objectives

Core Objectives

Objective Number	Objective Statement	Data Source
AOCBC-2030-01	Reduce the proportion of severe and moderate joint pain among adults with provider-diagnosed arthritis	National Health Interview Survey (NHIS), CDC/NCHS
AOCBC-2030-02	Reduce the proportion of adults with provider-diagnosed arthritis who experience a limitation in activity due to arthritis or joint symptoms	National Health Interview Survey (NHIS), CDC/NCHS
AOCBC-2030-03	Reduce the proportion of adults with provider-diagnosed arthritis who are limited in their ability to work for pay due to arthritis	National Health Interview Survey (NHIS), CDC/NCHS
AOCBC-2030-04	Increase the proportion of adults with provider-diagnosed arthritis who receive health care provider counseling for physical activity or exercise	National Health Interview Survey (NHIS), CDC/NCHS
AOCBC-2030-05	Reduce the proportion of adults with osteoporosis	National Health and Nutrition Examination Survey (NHANES), CDC/NCHS
AOCBC-2030-06	Reduce hip fractures among older adults - aged 65 years and older	Linked CMS Medicare data (due to the discontinuation of NHDS; Placeholder data is CMS Medicare data from Dartmouth Atlas of Health Care)
AOCBC-2030-07	Reduce the prevalence of adults having high impact chronic pain	National Health Interview Survey (NHIS), CDC/NCHS

Developmental Objectives

Objective Number	Objective Statement
AOCBC-2030-D01	Increase self-management of high impact chronic pain
AOCBC-2030-D02	Reduce the impact of high impact chronic pain on family/significant others

4. BDBS (Blood Disorders and Blood Safety)

2 Core Objectives; 2 Developmental Objectives; 0 Research Objectives

Core Objectives

Objective Number	Objective Statement	Data Source
BDBS-2030-01	Reduce the proportion of persons with severe hemophilia who have more than four joint bleeds per year	Community Counts Registry for Bleeding Disorders Surveillance, CDC/NCBDDD and ATHN
BDBS-2030-02	Increase the proportion of Medicare beneficiaries with sickle cell disease who receive disease modifying therapies	Medicare Administrative Data, CMS

Developmental Objectives

Objective Number	Objective Statement
BDBS-2030-D01	Increase the proportion of persons who donate blood
BDBS-2030-D02	Increase the proportion of persons with von Willebrand disease (VWD) seen in specialty care centers who were diagnosed by 21 years of age

5. C (Cancer)

11 Core Objectives; 0 Developmental Objectives; 2 Research Objectives

Core Objectives

Objective Number	Objective Statement	Data Source
C-2030-01	Reduce the overall cancer death rate	National Vital Statistics System-Mortality (NVSS-M), CDC/NCHS; Bridged-race Population Estimates, CDC/NCHS and Census
C-2030-02	Reduce the lung cancer death rate	National Vital Statistics System-Mortality (NVSS-M), CDC/NCHS; Bridged-race Population Estimates, CDC/NCHS and Census
C-2030-03	Increase the proportion of adults who receive a lung cancer screening based on the most recent guidelines	National Health Interview Survey (NHIS), CDC/NCHS
C-2030-04	Reduce the female breast cancer death rate	National Vital Statistics System-Mortality (NVSS-M), CDC/NCHS; Bridged-race Population Estimates, CDC/NCHS and Census
C-2030-05	Increase the proportion of women who receive a breast cancer screening based on the most recent guidelines	National Health Interview Survey (NHIS), CDC/NCHS
C-2030-06	Reduce the colorectal cancer death rate	National Vital Statistics System-Mortality (NVSS-M), CDC/NCHS; Bridged-race Population Estimates, CDC/NCHS and Census
C-2030-07	Increase the proportion of adults who receive a colorectal cancer screening based on the most recent guidelines	National Health Interview Survey (NHIS), CDC/NCHS
C-2030-08	Reduce the prostate cancer death rate	National Vital Statistics System-Mortality (NVSS-M), CDC/NCHS; Bridged-race Population Estimates, CDC/NCHS and Census
C-2030-09	Increase the proportion of women who receive a cervical cancer screening based on the most recent guidelines	National Health Interview Survey (NHIS), CDC/NCHS
C-2030-10	Reduce the proportion of adolescents in grades 9 through 12 who report sunburn	Youth Risk Behavior Surveillance System (YRBSS), CDC/NCHHSTP

Objective Number	Objective Statement	Data Source
C-2030-11	Increase the proportion of cancer survivors who are living 5 years or longer after diagnosis	National Program of Cancer Registries (NPCR), CDC/NCCDPHP; Surveillance, Epidemiology, and End Results Program (SEER), NIH/NCI; Bridged-race Population Estimates, CDC/NCHS and Census

Research Objectives

Objective Number	Objective Statement
C-2030-R01	Increase the mental and physical health-related quality of life of cancer survivors
C-2030-R02	Increase the proportion of persons who are counseled or are engaged in shared decision-making with their providers for clinical preventive services to prevent cancer

6. CKD (Chronic Kidney Disease)

10 Core Objectives; 0 Developmental Objectives; 0 Research Objectives

Core Objectives

Objective Number	Objective Statement	Data Source
CKD-2030-01	Reduce the proportion of the U.S. adult population with chronic kidney disease	National Health and Nutrition Examination Survey (NHANES), CDC/NCHS
CKD-2030-02	Increase the proportion of adults with chronic kidney disease who know they have reduced kidney function	National Health and Nutrition Examination Survey (NHANES), CDC/NCHS
CKD-2030-03	Increase the proportion of Medicare beneficiaries aged 65 years or older who have a follow-up evaluation of their kidney function 3 months after a hospitalization with acute kidney injury	United States Renal Data System (USRDS), NIH/NIDDK
CKD-2030-04	Increase the proportion of Medicare beneficiaries aged 65 years or older with chronic kidney disease who receive medical evaluation with serum creatinine, lipids, and urine albumin tests	United States Renal Data System (USRDS), NIH/NIDDK
CKD-2030-05	Increase the proportion of adults with diabetes and chronic kidney disease who receive recommended medical treatment with angiotensin-converting enzyme (ACE) inhibitors or angiotensin II receptor blockers (ARBs)	National Health and Nutrition Examination Survey (NHANES), CDC/NCHS
CKD-2030-06	Reduce the proportion of adults with chronic kidney disease who have elevated blood pressure	National Health and Nutrition Examination Survey (NHANES), CDC/NCHS
CKD-2030-07	Reduce the rate of new cases of end-stage kidney disease	United States Renal Data System (USRDS), NIH/NIDDK; Population
CKD-2030-08	Reduce the proportion of adult hemodialysis patients who use catheters as the only mode of vascular access	United States Renal Data System (USRDS), NIH/NIDDK
CKD-2030-09	Increase the proportion of persons younger than 70 years receiving a kidney transplant within 3 years of initiating treatment for end-stage kidney disease	United States Renal Data System (USRDS), NIH/NIDDK
CKD-2030-10	Reduce the death rate for persons on dialysis	United States Renal Data System (USRDS),

7. D (Diabetes)

9 Core Objectives; 1 Developmental Objective; 0 Research Objectives

Core Objectives

Objective Number	Objective Statement	Data Source
D-2030-01	Reduce the annual number of new cases of diagnosed diabetes in the population	National Health Interview Survey (NHIS), CDC/NCHS
D-2030-02	Reduce the rate of all-cause mortality among adults with diagnosed diabetes	National Health Interview Survey (NHIS), CDC/NCHS; National Death Index (NDI),
D-2030-03	Reduce the rate of lower extremity amputations in adults with diagnosed diabetes	Healthcare Cost and Utilization Project - Nationwide Inpatient Sample (HCUP-NIS), AHRQ
D-2030-04	Reduce the proportion of adults with diagnosed diabetes with an A1c value greater than 9 percent	National Health and Nutrition Examination Survey (NHANES), CDC/NCHS
D-2030-05	Increase the proportion of adults with diabetes who have an annual eye exam	National Health Interview Survey (NHIS), CDC/NCHS
D-2030-06	Increase the proportion of adults with known diabetes who receive an annual urinary albumin test	United States Renal Data System (USRDS), NIH/NIDDK
D-2030-07	Increase the proportion of adults with diabetes using insulin who perform self-monitoring of blood glucose at least once daily	Behavioral Risk Factor Surveillance System (BRFSS), CDC/NCCDPHP
D-2030-08	Increase the proportion of persons with diagnosed diabetes who ever receive formal diabetes education	Behavioral Risk Factor Surveillance System (BRFSS), CDC/NCCDPHP
D-2030-09	Reduce the proportion of adults with undiagnosed prediabetes	National Health and Nutrition Examination Survey (NHANES), CDC/NCHS

Developmental Objectives

Objective Number	Objective Statement
D-2030-D01	Increase the proportion of eligible individuals completing CDC-recognized lifestyle change programs

8. DH (Disability and Health)

6 Core Objectives; 0 Developmental Objectives; 0 Research Objectives

Core Objectives

Objective Number	Objective Statement	Data Source
DH-2030-01	Increase the proportion of nationally-representative, population-based surveys that include in their core a standardized set of questions that identify people with disabilities	Assessment of nationally-representative, population-based surveys, CDC/NCBDDD
DH-2030-02	Reduce the proportion of adults with disabilities aged 18 years and older who experience delays in receiving primary and periodic preventive care due to cost	National Health Interview Survey (NHIS), CDC/NCHS
DH-2030-03	Increase the proportion of children and youth with disabilities who spend at least 80 percent of their time in regular education programs	Individuals with Disabilities Education Act data (IDEA data), ED/OSERS
DH-2030-04	Reduce the proportion of people with disabilities who receive long-term care services that live in congregate care residences with seven or more people	Residential Information Systems Project (RISP) Annual Survey of State Developmental Disability Agencies, University of Minnesota
DH-2030-05	Increase the proportion of all occupied homes and residential buildings that have visitable features	American Housing Survey, HUD and Census
DH-2030-06	Reduce the proportion of adults with disabilities aged 18 years and older who experience serious psychological distress	National Health Interview Survey (NHIS), CDC/NCHS

9. DIA (Dementias, including Alzheimer's Disease)

3 Core Objectives; 0 Developmental Objectives; 0 Research Objectives

Core Objectives

Objective Number	Objective Statement	Data Source
DIA-2030-01	Increase the proportion of adults aged 65 years and older with diagnosed Alzheimer's disease and other dementias, or their caregiver, who are aware of the diagnosis	Medicare Current Beneficiary Survey (MCBS), CMS
DIA-2030-02	Reduce the proportion of preventable hospitalizations in adults aged 65 years and older with diagnosed Alzheimer's disease and other dementias	Health and Retirement Study (HRS), University of Michigan
DIA-2030-03	Increase the proportion of adults aged 65 years and older with Subjective Cognitive Decline (SCD) who have discussed their confusion or memory loss with a health care professional	Behavioral Risk Factor Surveillance System (BRFSS), CDC/NCCDPHP

10. ECBP (Educational and Community-Based Programs)

1 Core Objective; 13 Developmental Objectives; 0 Research Objectives

Core Objectives

Objective Number	Objective Statement	Data Source
ECBP-2030-01	Increase the proportion of adolescents who participate in daily school physical education	Youth Risk Behavior Surveillance System (YRBSS), CDC/NCHHSTP

Developmental Objectives

Objective Number	Objective Statement
ECBP-2030-D01	Increase the percentage of middle and high schools that provide case management for chronic conditions
ECBP-2030-D02	Increase the proportion of worksites that offer employee health promotion program(s) to their employees
ECBP-2030-D03	Increase the proportion of worksites that offer a physical activity program(s) as part of an employee health promotion program
ECBP-2030-D04	Increase the proportion of worksites that offer a nutrition program as part of an employee health promotion program
ECBP-2030-D05	Increase the proportion of worksites that are covered by indoor worksite policies that prohibit smoking
ECBP-2030-D06	Increase the number of community-based organizations providing population-based primary prevention services
ECBP-2030-D07	Increase the proportion of academic institutions with health professions education programs whose prevention and population health curricula include interprofessional experiential training
ECBP-2030-D08	Increase the inclusion of core clinical prevention and population health content in medical schools
ECBP-2030-D09	Increase the inclusion of core clinical prevention and population health content in undergraduate nursing and graduate nurse practitioner training programs
ECBP-2030-D10	Increase the inclusion of core clinical prevention and population health content in physician assistant training
ECBP-2030-D11	Increase the inclusion of core clinical prevention and population health content in Doctor of Pharmacy (PharmD) granting colleges and schools of pharmacy
ECBP-2030-D12	Increase the inclusion of core clinical prevention and population health content in Doctor of Dental Surgery and/or Doctor of Dental Medicine granting colleges and schools of Dentistry
ECBP-2030-D13	Increase the proportion of schools that do not sell less healthy foods

11. EH (Environmental Health)

15 Core Objectives; 0 Developmental Objectives; 0 Research Objectives

Core Objectives

Objective Number	Objective Statement	Data Source
EH-2030-01	Reduce the number of days people are exposed to unhealthy air	Air Quality System (AQS), EPA
EH-2030-02	Increase trips to work made by mass transit	American Community Survey (ACS), Census
EH-2030-03	Increase the proportion of persons who telecommute	American Community Survey (ACS), Census
EH-2030-04	Increase the proportion of persons served by community water systems who receive a supply of drinking water that meets the regulations of the Safe Drinking Water Act	Safe Drinking Water Information System (SDWIS); EPA/OW
EH-2030-05	Reduce blood lead level in children aged 1–5 years	National Health and Nutrition Examination Survey (NHANES), CDC/NCHS
EH-2030-06	Minimize the risks to human health and the environment posed by hazardous sites	Comprehensive Environmental Response and Cleanup Information System (CERCLIS),
EH-2030-07	Reduce the amount of toxic pollutants released into the environment	Toxics Release Inventory (TRI), EPA
EH-2030-08	Reduce exposure to arsenic in the population, as measured by blood or urine concentrations of the substance or its metabolites	National Report on Human Exposure to Environmental Chemicals, CDC/NCEH
EH-2030-09	Reduce exposure to lead in the population, as measured by blood or urine concentrations of the substance or its metabolites	National Report on Human Exposure to Environmental Chemicals, CDC/NCEH
EH-2030-10	Reduce exposure to mercury among children aged 1 to 5 years, as measured by blood or urine concentrations of the substance or its metabolites	National Report on Human Exposure to Environmental Chemicals, CDC/NCEH
EH-2030-11	Reduce exposure to bisphenol A in the population, as measured by blood or urine concentrations of the substance or its metabolites	National Report on Human Exposure to Environmental Chemicals, CDC/NCEH
EH-2030-12	Reduce exposure to perchlorate in the population, as measured by blood or urine concentrations of the substance or its metabolites	National Report on Human Exposure to Environmental Chemicals, CDC/NCEH
EH-2030-13	Increase the number of states, territories, tribes, and the District of Columbia that monitor diseases or conditions that can be caused by exposure to lead poisoning	State Reportable Conditions Data Inventory, Council of State and Territorial Epidemiologists (CSTE)

Objective Number	Objective Statement	Data Source
EH-2030-14	Increase the number of states, territories, tribes, and the District of Columbia that monitor diseases or conditions that can be caused by exposure to mercury poisoning	State Reportable Conditions Data Inventory, Council of State and Territorial Epidemiologists (CSTE)
EH-2030-15	Increase the number of states, territories, tribes, and the District of Columbia that monitor diseases or conditions that can be caused by exposure to arsenic poisoning	State Reportable Conditions Data Inventory, Council of State and Territorial Epidemiologists (CSTE)

12. EMC (Early and Middle Childhood)

4 Core Objectives; 2 Developmental Objectives; 0 Research Objectives

Core Objectives

Objective Number	Objective Statement	Data Source
EMC-2030-01	Increase the proportion of children aged 6-17 years who communicate positively with their parents	National Survey of Children's Health (NSCH), HRSA/MCHB
EMC-2030-02	Increase the proportion of young children whose parents read to them	National Survey of Children's Health (NSCH), HRSA/MCHB
EMC-2030-03	Increase the proportion of children who get sufficient sleep	National Survey of Children's Health (NSCH), HRSA/MCHB
EMC-2030-04	Increase the proportion of children aged 4-17 years with ADHD who receive any age-specific recommended treatment, including medication and/or behavioral therapy	National Survey of Children's Health (NSCH), HRSA/MCHB

Developmental Objectives

Objective Number	Objective Statement
EMC-2030-D01	Increase the number of children who are developmentally on track and ready for school
EMC-2030-D02	Reduce the number of children who experience exclusionary discipline in preschool

13. FP (Family Planning)

11 Core Objectives; 1 Developmental Objective; 0 Research Objectives

Core Objectives

Objective Number	Objective Statement	Data Source
FP-2030-01	Reduce the proportion of pregnancies that are unintended	National Survey of Family Growth (NSFG), CDC/NCHS; National Vital Statistics System-Natality (NVSS-N), CDC/NCHS; Abortion Surveillance Data, CDC/NCCDPHP; Guttmacher Institute Abortion Provider Census (APC), Guttmacher Institute; Guttmacher Institute Abortion Patient Survey (APS), Guttmacher Institute
FP-2030-02	Reduce the proportion of pregnancies conceived within 18 months of a previous birth	National Survey of Family Growth (NSFG), CDC/NCHS
FP-2030-03	Reduce pregnancies among adolescent females aged 15 to 19 years	National Vital Statistics System-Natality (NVSS-N), CDC/NCHS; Surveillance Data for Abortion, CDC/NCCDPHP; Guttmacher Institute Abortion Provider Census (ACS), Guttmacher Institute; Population Estimates, Census
FP-2030-04	Increase the proportion of adolescents aged 15-17 years who have never had sexual intercourse	National Survey of Family Growth (NSFG), CDC/NCHS
FP-2030-05	Increase the proportion of sexually active females aged 15 to 19 years who use a condom and hormonal or intrauterine contraception at last intercourse	National Survey of Family Growth (NSFG), CDC/NCHS
FP-2030-06	Increase the proportion of sexually active males aged 15 to 19 years who used a condom at last intercourse	National Survey of Family Growth (NSFG), CDC/NCHS
FP-2030-07	Increase the proportion of sexually active adolescents aged 15 to 19 years who use any method of contraception at first intercourse	National Survey of Family Growth (NSFG), CDC/NCHS
FP-2030-08	Increase the proportion of female adolescents who received formal instruction on delayed sex, birth control methods, HIV/AIDS prevention, and sexually transmitted diseases before they were 18	National Survey of Family Growth (NSFG), CDC/NCHS

Objective Number	Objective Statement	Data Source
FP-2030-09	Increase the proportion of females in need of publicly supported contraceptive services and supplies who receive those services and supplies	National Survey of Family Growth (NSFG), CDC/NCHS; Guttmacher Institute Abortion Provider Census (APC), Guttmacher Institute
FP-2030-10	Increase the proportion of females aged 20 to 44 years at risk of unintended pregnancy who use most effective or moderately effective methods of contraception	National Survey of Family Growth (NSFG), CDC/NCHS
FP-2030-11	Increase the proportion of adolescent females aged 15 to 19 at risk of unintended pregnancy who use most effective or moderately effective methods of contraception	National Survey of Family Growth (NSFG), CDC/NCHS

Developmental Objectives

Objective Number	Objective Statement
FP-2030-D01	Increase the proportion of publicly funded family planning clinics that offer the full range of reversible contraceptive methods onsite

14. FS (Food Safety)

12 Core Objectives; 7 Developmental Objectives; 0 Research Objectives

Core Objectives

Objective Number	Objective Statement	Data Source
FS-2030-01	Reduce the incidence of laboratory-diagnosed, domestically-acquired Campylobacter infections	Foodborne Diseases Active Surveillance Network (FoodNet), CDC/NCEZID
FS-2030-02	Reduce the incidence of laboratory-diagnosed, domestically-acquired Shiga toxin-producing Escherichia coli (STEC) infections	Foodborne Diseases Active Surveillance Network (FoodNet), CDC/NCEZID
FS-2030-03	Reduce the incidence of laboratory-diagnosed, domestically-acquired Listeria monocytogenes infections	Foodborne Diseases Active Surveillance Network (FoodNet), CDC/NCEZID
FS-2030-04	Reduce the incidence of laboratory-diagnosed, domestically-acquired Salmonella infections	Foodborne Diseases Active Surveillance Network (FoodNet), CDC/NCEZID
FS-2030-05	Prevent an increase in the proportion of nontyphoidal Salmonella infections in humans that are resistant to three or more drug classes	National Antimicrobial Resistance Monitoring System for Enteric Bacteria (NARMS), CDC/NCEZID
FS-2030-06	Prevent an increase in the proportion of domestically-acquired Campylobacter jejuni infections in humans that are resistant to macrolides	National Antimicrobial Resistance Monitoring System for Enteric Bacteria (NARMS), CDC/NCEZID; Foodborne Diseases Active Surveillance Network (FoodNet), CDC/NCEZID
FS-2030-07	Increase the proportion of consumers who follow the key food safety practice of "Clean: wash hands and surfaces often"	Food Safety Survey, FDA
FS-2030-08	Increase the proportion of consumers who follow the key food safety practice of "Cook: cook to the safe internal temperature"	Food Safety Survey, FDA
FS-2030-09	Increase the proportion of retail food store delis where food employees practice proper handwashing	Retail Food Risk Factor Studies, FDA/CFSAN
FS-2030-10	Increase the proportion of retail food store delis where food contact surfaces are properly cleaned and sanitized	Retail Food Risk Factor Studies, FDA/CFSAN
FS-2030-11	Increase the proportion of retail food store delis where foods requiring refrigeration are held at the proper temperature	Retail Food Risk Factor Studies, FDA/CFSAN
FS-2030-12	Increase the proportion of retail food store delis where foods displayed or stored hot are held at the proper temperature	Retail Food Risk Factor Studies, FDA/CFSAN

Developmental Objectives

Objective Number	Objective Statement
FS-2030-D01	Reduce the number of infections due to outbreaks of Shiga toxin-producing E. coli, or Campylobacter, Listeria or Salmonella species associated with beef
FS-2030-D02	Reduce the number of infections due to outbreaks of Shiga toxin-producing E. coli, or Campylobacter, Listeria or Salmonella species associated with dairy
FS-2030-D03	Reduce the number of infections due to outbreaks of Shiga toxin-producing E. coli , or Campylobacter, Listeria or Salmonella species associated with fruit and nuts
FS-2030-D04	Reduce the number of infections due to outbreaks of Shiga toxin-producing E. coli, or Campylobacter, Listeria or Salmonella species associated with leafy greens
FS-2030-D05	Reduce the number of infections due to outbreaks of Shiga toxin-producing E. coli, or Campylobacter, Listeria or Salmonella species associated with poultry
FS-2030-D06	Reduce the number of outbreaks of infections caused by Norovirus
FS-2030-D07	Reduce the number of food allergy reactions requiring emergency treatment

15. GH (Global Health)

1 Core Objective; 1 Developmental Objective; 1 Research Objective

Core Objectives

Objective Number	Objective Statement	Data Source
GH-2030-01	Increase the number of field epidemiologists trained globally by the Department of Health and Human Services	Global Health Security Report, CDC

Developmental Objectives

Objective Number	Objective Statement
GH-2030-D01	Increase the number of public health events of international importance monitored and reported

Research Objectives

Objective Number	Objective Statement
GH-2030-R01	Increase laboratory diagnostic testing capacity in countries and regionally through the Department of Health and Human Services

16. HAI (Healthcare-Associated Infections)

2 Core Objectives; 1 Developmental Objective; 0 Research Objectives

Core Objectives

Objective Number	Objective Statement	Data Source
HAI-2030-01	Reduce hospital-onset Clostridioides difficile infections	National Healthcare Safety Network (NHSN), CDC/NCEZID
HAI-2030-02	Reduce hospital-onset MRSA bacteremia	National Healthcare Safety Network (NHSN), CDC/NCEZID

Developmental Objectives

Objective Number	Objective Statement
HAI-2030-D01	Reduce inappropriate antibiotic use in outpatient settings

17. HC/HIT (Health Communication and Health Information Technology)

7 Core Objectives; 8 Developmental Objectives; 0 Research Objectives

Core Objectives

Objective Number	Objective Statement	Data Source
HC/HIT-2030-01	Increase the proportion of persons who report their health care provider always asked them to describe how they will follow instructions	Medical Expenditure Panel Survey (MEPS), AHRQ
HC/HIT-2030-02	Reduce the proportion of persons who report poor patient/provider communication (e.g., listening, explanations, disrespect, time)	Medical Expenditure Panel Survey (MEPS), AHRQ
HC/HIT-2030-03	Increase the proportion of persons who report that their health care providers always involved them in decisions about their health care as much as they wanted	Health Information National Trends Survey (HINTS), NIH/NCI
HC/HIT-2030-04	Increase proportion of persons who use health information technology (HIT) to track health care data or communicate with providers	Health Information National Trends Survey (HINTS), NIH/NCI
HC/HIT-2030-05	Increase the proportion of persons with broadband access to the Internet	Health Information National Trends Survey (HINTS), NIH/NCI
HC/HIT-2030-06	Increase the proportion of persons offered online access to their medical record	Health Information National Trends Survey (HINTS), NIH/NCI
HC/HIT-2030-07	Increase the proportion of adults who report having social support (having friends or family members that they talk to about their	Health Information National Trends Survey (HINTS), NIH/NCI

Developmental Objectives

Objective Number	Objective Statement
HC/HIT-2030-D01	Increase the proportion of persons who have access to quality (reliable and easy to use) digital health tools and information
HC/HIT-2030-D02	Increase the number of state health departments that report using social marketing in health promotion and disease prevention programs

Objective Number	Objective Statement
HC/HIT-2030-D03	Increase the proportion of crisis and emergency risk messages embedded in print and broadcast news stories that present complete information (i.e., what is known, what is not known, and how or why the event happened)
HC/HIT-2030-D04	Increase the proportion of crisis and emergency risk messages embedded in print and broadcast news stories that promote steps the reader or viewer can take to reduce their personal health threat
HC/HIT-2030-D05	Increase the proportion of crisis and emergency risk messages embedded in print and broadcast news stories that demonstrate engagement (i.e., express empathy, accountability, and commitment)
HC/HIT-2030-D06	Increase the percentage of clinicians that can send, receive, find, and integrate electronic health information from outside sources
HC/HIT-2030-D07	Increase the percentage of clinicians that have necessary information electronically available at the point of care
HC/HIT-2030-D08	Increase the proportion of persons that can view, download, and transmit their electronic health information

18. HDS (Heart Disease and Stroke)

9 Core Objectives; 7 Developmental Objectives; 0 Research Objectives

Core Objectives

Objective Number	Objective Statement	Data Source
HDS-2030-01	Increase overall cardiovascular health in U.S. adults	National Health and Nutrition Examination Survey (NHANES), CDC/NCHS
HDS-2030-02	Reduce coronary heart disease deaths	National Vital Statistics System-Mortality (NVSS-M), CDC/NCHS; Bridged-race Population Estimates, CDC/NCHS and Census
HDS-2030-03	Reduce stroke deaths	National Vital Statistics System-Mortality (NVSS-M), CDC/NCHS; Bridged-race Population Estimates, CDC/NCHS and Census
HDS-2030-04	Reduce the proportion of adults with hypertension	National Health and Nutrition Examination Survey (NHANES), CDC/NCHS
HDS-2030-05	Reduce the mean total blood cholesterol levels among adults	National Health and Nutrition Examination Survey (NHANES), CDC/NCHS
HDS-2030-06	Increase the proportion of adults with hypertension whose blood pressure is under control	National Health and Nutrition Examination Survey (NHANES), CDC/NCHS
HDS-2030-07	Increase the proportion of adults with a history of cardiovascular disease who are using aspirin therapy to prevent recurrent cardiovascular events	National Health and Nutrition Examination Survey (NHANES), CDC/NCHS
HDS-2030-08	Reduce hospitalizations among adults with heart failure as the principal diagnosis	Healthcare Cost and Utilization Project - Nationwide Inpatient Sample (HCUP-NIS), AHRQ; Population Estimates, Census
HDS-2030-09	Increase the treatment of blood cholesterol among eligible adults	National Health and Nutrition Examination Survey (NHANES), CDC/NCHS

Developmental Objectives

Objective Number	Objective Statement
HDS-2030-D01	Increase the proportion of eligible patients with heart attacks who receive fibrinolytic therapy within 30 minutes of hospital arrival
HDS-2030-D02	Increase the proportion of eligible patients with heart attacks who receive percutaneous intervention (PCI) within 90 minutes of hospital arrival
HDS-2030-D03	Increase the proportion of eligible patients with strokes who receive acute intravenous reperfusion therapy within 3 hours from symptom onset
HDS-2030-D04	Increase the proportion of adult heart attack survivors who are referred to a cardiac rehabilitation program at discharge
HDS-2030-D05	Increase the proportion of adult stroke survivors who participate in rehabilitation services
HDS-2030-D06	Increase the proportion of adults who have had their risk for developing atherosclerotic cardiovascular disease (ACVD) assessed
HDS-2030-D07	Increase the proportion of eligible patients with strokes who receive mechanical thrombectomy within 16 hours from symptom onset

19. HIV

6 Core Objectives; 0 Developmental Objectives; 0 Research Objectives

Core Objectives

Objective Number	Objective Statement	Data Source
HIV-2030-01	Reduce the number of new HIV infections among adolescents and adults, 13 years and older	National HIV Surveillance System (NHSS), CDC/NCHHSTP
HIV-2030-02	Increase the proportion of persons 13 years and older who know their HIV status	National HIV Surveillance System (NHSS), CDC/NCHHSTP
HIV-2030-03	Reduce the number of new HIV diagnoses among persons of all ages	National HIV Surveillance System (NHSS), CDC/NCHHSTP
HIV-2030-04	Increase the percentage of persons 13 years and older with newly diagnosed HIV infection linked to HIV medical care within one	National HIV Surveillance System (NHSS), CDC/NCHHSTP
HIV-2030-05	Increase the percentage of persons 13 years and older with diagnosed HIV infection who are virally suppressed	National HIV Surveillance System (NHSS), CDC/NCHHSTP
HIV-2030-06	Reduce rate of newly diagnosed perinatally acquired HIV infections	National HIV Surveillance System (NHSS), CDC/NCHHSTP; National Vital Statistics System (NVSS), CDC/NCHS

20. HOSCD (Hearing and Other Sensory or Communication Disorders)

12 Core Objectives; 0 Developmental Objectives; 0 Research Objectives

Core Objectives

Objective Number	Objective Statement	Data Source
HOSCD-2030-01	Increase the proportion of newborns who are screened for hearing loss by no later than age 1 month	Early Hearing Detection and Intervention (EHDI) Hearing Screening and Follow-up Survey (EHDI HSFS), CDC/NCBDDD
HOSCD-2030-02	Increase the proportion of infants who did not pass the hearing screening test that receive diagnostic audiologic evaluation for hearing loss no later than age 3 months	Early Hearing Detection and Intervention (EHDI) Hearing Screening and Follow-up Survey (EHDI HSFS), CDC/NCBDDD
HOSCD-2030-03	Increase the proportion of infants with confirmed hearing loss who are enrolled for intervention services no later than age 6 months	Early Hearing Detection and Intervention (EHDI) Hearing Screening and Follow-up Survey (EHDI HSFS), CDC/NCBDDD
HOSCD-2030-04	Reduce frequent ear infections (otitis media) in children	National Health Interview Survey (NHIS), CDC/NCHS
HOSCD-2030-05	Increase the proportion of adults with hearing loss who use a hearing aid	National Health Interview Survey (NHIS), CDC/NCHS
HOSCD-2030-06	Increase the proportion of adults who have had a hearing examination within the past 5 years	National Health and Nutrition Examination Survey (NHANES), CDC/NCHS
HOSCD-2030-07	Increase the proportion of adults who use hearing protection devices (earplugs, earmuffs) when exposed to loud sounds or music	National Health and Nutrition Examination Survey (NHANES), CDC/NCHS
HOSCD-2030-08	Reduce the proportion of adults who have hearing loss due to noise exposure	National Health and Nutrition Examination Survey (NHANES), CDC/NCHS
HOSCD-2030-09	Increase the proportion of adults with onset of bothersome tinnitus in the past 5 years who have seen a health care specialist	National Health Interview Survey (NHIS), CDC/NCHS
HOSCD-2030-10	Increase the proportion of adults with moderate to severe balance or dizziness problems who have seen or been referred to a health care specialist for evaluation and treatment	National Health Interview Survey (NHIS), CDC/NCHS
HOSCD-2030-11	Increase the proportion of adults with smell or taste disorders who have ever seen a health care provider about their disorder	National Health and Nutrition Examination Survey (NHANES), CDC/NCHS

Objective Number	Objective Statement	Data Source
HOSCD-2030-12	Increase the proportion of children with communication disorders of voice, speech, or language who have seen a health care specialist for evaluation or treatment in the past 12 months	National Health Interview Survey (NHIS), CDC/NCHS

21. IID (Immunization and Infectious Diseases)

16 Core Objectives; 1 Developmental Objective; 0 Research Objectives

Core Objectives

Objective Number	Objective Statement	Data Source
IID-2030-01	Reduce the rate of hepatitis A	National Notifiable Diseases Surveillance System (NNDSS), CDC/PHSIPO; Bridged-race Population Estimates, CDC/NCHS and Census
IID-2030-02	Reduce the rate of acute hepatitis B	National Notifiable Diseases Surveillance System (NNDSS), CDC/PHSIPO; Bridged-race Population Estimates, CDC/NCHS and Census
IID-2030-03	Reduce the rate of acute hepatitis C	National Notifiable Diseases Surveillance System (NNDSS), CDC/PHSIPO; Bridged-race Population Estimates, CDC/NCHS and Census
IID-2030-04	Increase the proportion of persons aware they have chronic hepatitis B	National Health and Nutrition Examination Survey (NHANES), CDC/NCHS
IID-2030-05	Increase the proportion of persons aware they have chronic hepatitis C	National Health and Nutrition Examination Survey (NHANES), CDC/NCHS
IID-2030-06	Reduce the rate of deaths with hepatitis C as the underlying or a contributing cause	National Vital Statistics System-Mortality (NVSS-M), CDC/NCHS; Bridged-race Population Estimates, CDC/NCHS and Census
IID-2030-07	Reduce tuberculosis (TB)	National Tuberculosis Surveillance System (NTSS), CDC/NCHHSTP; Bridged-race Population Estimates, CDC/NCHS and Census
IID-2030-08	Reduce cases of pertussis among children under 1 year of age	National Notifiable Diseases Surveillance System (NNDSS), CDC/PHSIPO
IID-2030-09	Increase the vaccination coverage level of 4 doses of the diphtheria-tetanus-acellular pertussis (DTaP) vaccine among children by age 2 years	National Immunization Survey-Child (NIS-Child), CDC/NCIRD and CDC/NCHS
IID-2030-10	Maintain an effective vaccination coverage level of 1 dose of measles- mumps-rubella vaccine (MMR) among children by age 2	National Immunization Survey-Child (NIS-Child), CDC/NCIRD and CDC/NCHS

Objective Number	Objective Statement	Data Source
IID-2030-11	Reduce the percentage of children in the U.S. who receive 0 doses of recommended vaccines by age 2 years	National Immunization Survey-Child (NIS-Child), CDC/NCIRD and CDC/NCHS
IID-2030-12	Increase the percentage of adolescents aged 13 through 15 years who receive recommended doses of human papillomavirus (HPV) vaccine	National Immunization Survey-Teen (NIS-Teen), CDC/NCIRD and CDC/NCHS
IID-2030-13	Increase the percentage of noninstitutionalized persons aged 6 months and older who are vaccinated annually against seasonal influenza	National Health Interview Survey (NHIS), CDC/NCHS
IID-2030-14	Reduce infections due to human papillomavirus (HPV) types prevented by the 9 valent vaccine	National Health and Nutrition Examination Survey (NHANES), CDC/NCHS
IID-2030-15	Maintain elimination of measles, rubella, congenital rubella syndrome (CRS), and acute paralytic poliomyelitis	National Notifiable Diseases Surveillance System (NNDSS), CDC/PHSIPO
IID-2030-16	Maintain the vaccination coverage level of 2 doses of measles-mumps- rubella (MMR) vaccine for children in kindergarten	Annual School Assessment Reports, CDC/NCIRD

Developmental Objectives

Objective Number	Objective Statement
IID-2030-D01	Increase the percentage of pregnant women who receive one dose of Tdap during pregnancy

22. IVP (Injury and Violence Prevention)

18 Core Objectives; 4 Developmental Objectives; 0 Research Objectives

Core Objectives

Objective Number	Objective Statement	Data Source
IVP-2030-01	Reduce fatal injuries	National Vital Statistics System-Mortality (NVSS-M), CDC/NCHS; Bridged-race Population Estimates, CDC/NCHS and Census
IVP-2030-02	Reduce fatal traumatic brain injuries	National Vital Statistics System-Mortality (NVSS-M), CDC/NCHS; Bridged-race Population Estimates, CDC/NCHS and Census
IVP-2030-03	Reduce unintentional injury deaths	National Vital Statistics System-Mortality (NVSS-M), CDC/NCHS; Bridged-race Population Estimates, CDC/NCHS and Census
IVP-2030-04	Reduce emergency department visits for nonfatal unintentional injuries	National Electronic Injury Surveillance System-All Injury Program (NEISS-AIP), CDC/NCIPC and CPSC; Bridged-race Population Estimates, CDC/NCHS and Census
IVP-2030-05	Reduce motor vehicle crash-related deaths	National Vital Statistics System-Mortality (NVSS-M), CDC/NCHS; Bridged-race Population Estimates, CDC/NCHS and Census
IVP-2030-06	Reduce the proportion of passenger vehicle occupant deaths that were known unrestrained	Fatality Analysis Reporting System (FARS), DOT/NHTSA
IVP-2030-07	Reduce fall-related deaths among adults aged 65 years and older	National Vital Statistics System-Mortality (NVSS-M), CDC/NCHS; Bridged-race Population Estimates, CDC/NCHS and Census
IVP-2030-08	Reduce homicides	Bridged-race Population Estimates, CDC/NCHS and Census; National Vital Statistics System-Mortality (NVSS-M), CDC/NCHS

Objective Number	Objective Statement	Data Source
IVP-2030-09	Reduce nonfatal physical assault injuries	Bridged-race Population Estimates, CDC/NCHS and Census; National Electronic Injury Surveillance System-All Injury Program (NEISS-AIP), CDC/NCIPC and CPSC
IVP-2030-10	Reduce physical fighting among adolescents	Youth Risk Behavior Surveillance System (YRBSS), CDC/NCHHSTP
IVP-2030-11	Reduce gun carrying among adolescents	Youth Risk Behavior Surveillance System (YRBSS), CDC/NCHHSTP
IVP-2030-12	Reduce firearm-related deaths	Bridged-race Population Estimates, CDC/NCHS and Census; National Vital Statistics System-Mortality (NVSS-M), CDC/NCHS
IVP-2030-13	Reduce nonfatal firearm-related injuries	Bridged-race Population Estimates, CDC/NCHS and Census; National Electronic Injury Surveillance System (NEISS), CDC/NCIPC and CPSC
IVP-2030-14	Reduce child abuse and neglect deaths	National Child Abuse and Neglect Data System (NCANDS), ACF; Population Estimates,
IVP-2030-15	Reduce nonfatal child abuse and neglect	National Child Abuse and Neglect Data System (NCANDS), ACF; Population Estimates,
IVP-2030-16	Reduce adolescent sexual violence by anyone	Youth Risk Behavior Surveillance System (YRBSS), CDC/NCHHSTP
IVP-2030-17	Reduce adolescent dating violence (sexual or physical)	Youth Risk Behavior Surveillance System (YRBSS), CDC/NCHHSTP
IVP-2030-18	Reduce nonfatal intentional self-harm injuries	Bridged-race Population Estimates, CDC/NCHS and Census; National Electronic Injury Surveillance System-All Injury Program (NEISS-AIP), CDC/NCIPC and CPSC

Developmental Objectives

Objective Number	Objective Statement
IVP-2030-D01	Increase the number of states where external causes of deaths among children are reviewed by a child fatality review team
IVP-2030-D02	Increase the number of states where sudden and unexpected deaths to infants are reviewed by a child fatality review team
IVP-2030-D03	Reduce intimate partner violence (i.e., contact sexual violence, physical violence, and stalking) across the lifespan
IVP-2030-D04	Reduce contact sexual violence by anyone across the lifespan

23. LGBT (Lesbian, Gay, Bisexual, and Transgender Health)

7 Core Objectives; 0 Developmental Objectives; 0 Research Objectives

Core Objectives

Objective Number	Objective Statement	Data Source
LGBT-2030-01	Increase the number of nationally representative, population-based surveys that collect data on (or for) lesbian, gay and bisexual populations	Healthy People 2030 Database (DATA2030), CDC/NCHS
LGBT-2030-02	Increase the number of nationally representative, population-based surveys that collect data on (or for) transgender populations	Healthy People 2030 Database (DATA2030), CDC/NCHS
LGBT-2030-03	Increase the number of states, territories, and the District of Columbia that include questions on sexual orientation and gender identity in the Behavioral Risk Factor Surveillance System (BRFSS)	Behavioral Risk Factor Surveillance System (BRFSS), CDC/NCCDPHP
LGBT-2030-04	Increase the number of states, territories, and the District of Columbia that use the standard module on sexual orientation and gender identity in the Behavioral Risk Factor Surveillance System (BRFSS)	Behavioral Risk Factor Surveillance System (BRFSS), CDC/NCCDPHP
LGBT-2030-05	Reduce bullying of sexual minority (gay, lesbian, bisexual, or not sure) high-school students	Youth Risk Behavior Surveillance System (YRBSS), CDC/NCHHSTP
LGBT-2030-06	Reduce suicidal ideation among sexual minority high school students, including those who seriously considered suicide, made a plan, or made an attempt in the past year	Youth Risk Behavior Surveillance System (YRBSS), CDC/NCHHSTP
LGBT-2030-07	Reduce proportion of sexual minority youth in high school who have ever used illicit drugs	Youth Risk Behavior Surveillance System (YRBSS), CDC/NCHHSTP

24. MHMD (Mental Health and Mental Disorders)

8 Core Objectives; 1 Developmental Objective; 1 Research Objective

Core Objectives

Objective Number	Objective Statement	Data Source
MHMD-2030-01	Reduce the suicide rate	National Vital Statistics System-Mortality (NVSS-M), CDC/NCHS; Bridged-race Population Estimates, CDC/NCHS and Census
MHMD-2030-02	Reduce suicide attempts by adolescents	Youth Risk Behavior Surveillance System (YRBSS), CDC/NCHHSTP
MHMD-2030-03	Increase the proportion of children with mental health problems who receive treatment	National Health Interview Survey (NHIS), CDC/NCHS
MHMD-2030-04	Increase the proportion of adults with serious mental illness (SMI) who receive treatment	National Survey on Drug Use and Health (NSDUH), SAMHSA
MHMD-2030-05	Increase the proportion of adults with major depressive episodes (MDEs) who receive treatment	National Survey on Drug Use and Health (NSDUH), SAMHSA
MHMD-2030-06	Increase the proportion of adolescents with major depressive episodes (MDEs) who receive treatment	National Survey on Drug Use and Health (NSDUH), SAMHSA
MHMD-2030-07	Increase the proportion of persons with co-occurring substance use disorders and mental disorders who received treatment for both disorders	National Survey on Drug Use and Health (NSDUH), SAMHSA
MHMD-2030-08	Increase the proportion of primary care physician office visits where adolescents and adults are screened for depression	National Ambulatory Medical Care Survey (NAMCS), CDC/NCHS

Developmental Objectives

Objective Number	Objective Statement
MHMD-2030-D01	Increase number of youth with serious emotional disturbance (SED) who are identified and receive treatment

Research Objectives

Objective Number	Objective Statement
MHMD-2030-R01	Increase the proportion of homeless adults with mental health problems who receive mental health services

25. MICH (Maternal, Infant, and Child Health)

19 Core Objectives; 3 Developmental Objectives; 0 Research Objectives

Core Objectives

Objective Number	Objective Statement	Data Source
MICH-2030-01	Reduce the rate of fetal deaths at 20 or more weeks of gestation	National Vital Statistics System-Fetal Death (NVSS- FD), CDC/NCHS; National Vital Statistics System- Natality (NVSS-N),
MICH-2030-02	Reduce the rate of all infant deaths (within 1 year)	Linked Birth/Infant Death Data Set, CDC/NCHS
MICH-2030-03	Reduce the rate of deaths among children and adolescents aged 1 to 19 years	National Vital Statistics System-Mortality (NVSS-M), CDC/NCHS; Bridged-race Population Estimates, CDC/NCHS and Census
MICH-2030-04	Reduce maternal deaths	National Vital Statistics System-Mortality (NVSS-M), CDC/NCHS; National Vital Statistics System-Natality (NVSS-N), CDC/NCHS
MICH-2030-05	Reduce severe maternal complications of pregnancy identified during labor and delivery hospitalizations	Healthcare Cost and Utilization Project - Nationwide Inpatient Sample (HCUP-NIS), AHRQ
MICH-2030-06	Reduce cesarean births among low-risk women with no prior births	National Vital Statistics System-Natality (NVSS-N), CDC/NCHS
MICH-2030-07	Reduce preterm births	National Vital Statistics System-Natality (NVSS-N), CDC/NCHS
MICH-2030-08	Increase the proportion of pregnant women who receive early and adequate prenatal care	National Vital Statistics System-Natality (NVSS-N), CDC/NCHS
MICH-2030-09	Increase abstinence from alcohol among pregnant women	National Survey on Drug Use and Health (NSDUH), SAMHSA
MICH-2030-10	Increase abstinence from cigarette smoking among pregnant women	National Vital Statistics System-Mortality (NVSS-M), CDC/NCHS; National Vital Statistics System-Natality (NVSS-N), CDC/NCHS
MICH-2030-11	Increase abstinence from illicit drugs among pregnant women	National Survey on Drug Use and Health (NSDUH), SAMHSA

Objective Number	Objective Statement	Data Source
MICH-2030-12	Increase the proportion of women of childbearing age who have optimal red blood cell folate concentrations	National Health and Nutrition Examination Survey (NHANES), CDC/NCHS
MICH-2030-13	Increase the proportion of women delivering a live birth who had a healthy weight prior to pregnancy	National Vital Statistics System-Natality (NVSS-N), CDC/NCHS
MICH-2030-14	Increase the proportion of infants who are put to sleep on their backs	Pregnancy Risk Assessment Monitoring System (PRAMS), CDC/NCCDPHP; California's Maternal and Infant Health Assessment (MIHA), CDPH
MICH-2030-15	Increase the proportion of infants who are breastfed exclusively through 6 months	National Immunization Survey (NIS), CDC/NCIRD and CDC/NCHS
MICH-2030-16	Increase the proportion of children (aged 9-35 months) who have completed a developmental screening	National Survey of Children's Health (NSCH), HRSA/MCHB
MICH-2030-17	Increase the proportion of children with autism spectrum disorder (ASD) enrolled in special services by 48 months of age	National Survey of Children's Health (NSCH), HRSA/MCHB
MICH-2030-18	Increase the proportion of children who have access to a medical home	National Survey of Children's Health (NSCH), HRSA/MCHB
MICH-2030-19	Increase the proportion of children with special health care needs who receive care in a family-centered, comprehensive, and coordinated system	National Survey of Children's Health (NSCH), HRSA/MCHB

Developmental Objectives

Objective Number	Objective Statement
MICH-2030-D01	Increase the percentage of women who are screened for postpartum depression at their postpartum checkup
MICH-2030-D02	Reduce the proportion of pregnant women who use illicit opioid pain relievers during pregnancy
MICH-2030-D03	Increase the proportion of infants who are put to sleep in a safe sleep environment

26. MPS (Medical Product Safety)

2 Core Objectives; 3 Developmental Objectives; 0 Research Objectives

Core Objectives

Objective	Objective Statement	Data Source
MPS-2030-01	Increase the proportion of medical-surgical hospitals that report adverse drug events	National Survey of Pharmacy Practice in Hospital Care Settings, ASHP
MPS-2030-02	Reduce emergency department visits for medication overdoses among children less than 5 years of age	Bridged-race Population Estimates, CDC/NCHS and Census; National Electronic Injury Surveillance System-Cooperative Adverse Drug Event Surveillance Project (NEISS-CADES), CDC and CPSC and FDA

Developmental Objectives

Objective Number	Objective Statement
MPS-2030-D01	Reduce emergency department visits for overdoses from oral anticoagulants
MPS-2030-D02	Reduce emergency department visits for overdoses from insulin
MPS-2030-D03	Increase the usage of medical products (drugs and biologics) associated with companion diagnostics

27. NWS (Nutrition and Weight Status)

16 Core Objectives; 0 Developmental Objectives; 0 Research Objectives

Core Objectives

Objective Number	Objective Statement	Data Source
NWS-2030-01	Reduce household food insecurity and in doing so reduce hunger	Current Population Survey Food Security Supplement (CPS-FSS), Census and USDA/ERS
NWS-2030-02	Reduce the proportion of adults who have obesity	National Health and Nutrition Examination Survey (NHANES), CDC/NCHS
NWS-2030-03	Reduce the proportion of children and adolescents aged 2 to 19 years who have obesity	National Health and Nutrition Examination Survey (NHANES), CDC/NCHS
NWS-2030-04	Increase the proportion of physician office visits made by adult patients who have obesity that include counseling or education related to weight reduction, nutrition, or physical activity	National Ambulatory Medical Care Survey (NAMCS), CDC/NCHS
NWS-2030-05	Increase consumption of fruits in the population aged 2 years and older	National Health and Nutrition Examination Survey (NHANES), CDC/NCHS
NWS-2030-06	Increase consumption of total vegetables in the population aged 2 years and older	National Health and Nutrition Examination Survey (NHANES), CDC/NCHS
NWS-2030-07	Increase consumption of dark green vegetables, red and orange vegetables, and beans and peas in the population aged 2 years and older	National Health and Nutrition Examination Survey (NHANES), CDC/NCHS
NWS-2030-08	Increase consumption of whole grains in the population aged 2 years and older	National Health and Nutrition Examination Survey (NHANES), CDC/NCHS
NWS-2030-09	Reduce consumption of calories from added sugars in the population aged 2 years and older	National Health and Nutrition Examination Survey (NHANES), CDC/NCHS
NWS-2030-10	Reduce consumption of saturated fat in the population aged 2 years and older	National Health and Nutrition Examination Survey (NHANES), CDC/NCHS
NWS-2030-11	Reduce consumption of sodium in the population aged 2 years and older	National Health and Nutrition Examination Survey (NHANES), CDC/NCHS
NWS-2030-12	Increase consumption of calcium in the population aged 2 years and older	National Health and Nutrition Examination Survey (NHANES), CDC/NCHS

Objective Number	Objective Statement	Data Source
NWS-2030-13	Increase consumption of potassium in the population aged 2 years and older	National Health and Nutrition Examination Survey (NHANES), CDC/NCHS
NWS-2030-14	Increase consumption of vitamin D in the population aged 2 years and older	National Health and Nutrition Examination Survey (NHANES), CDC/NCHS
NWS-2030-15	Reduce iron deficiency among children aged 1 to 2 years	National Health and Nutrition Examination Survey (NHANES), CDC/NCHS
NWS-2030-16	Reduce iron deficiency among females aged 12 to 49 years	National Health and Nutrition Examination Survey (NHANES), CDC/NCHS

28. OA (Older Adults)

7 Core Objectives; 0 Developmental Objectives; 0 Research Objectives

Core Objectives

Objective Number	Objective Statement	Data Source
OA-2030-01	Increase the proportion of older adults with reduced physical or cognitive function who engage in light, moderate, or vigorous leisure-time physical activities	National Health Interview Survey (NHIS), CDC/NCHS
OA-2030-02	Reduce the rate of pressure ulcer-related hospital admissions among older adults	Healthcare Cost and Utilization Project - Nationwide Inpatient Sample (HCUP-NIS), AHRQ
OA-2030-03	Reduce the rate of emergency department visits due to falls among older adults	Healthcare Cost and Utilization Project - Nationwide Emergency Department Sample (HCUP-NEDS),
OA-2030-04	Reduce the proportion of older adults who use inappropriate medications	Medical Expenditure Panel Survey (MEPS), AHRQ
OA-2030-05	Reduce the rate of hospital admissions for diabetes among older adults	Healthcare Cost and Utilization Project - Nationwide Inpatient Sample (HCUP-NIS), AHRQ
OA-2030-06	Reduce the rate of hospital admissions for pneumonia among older adults	Healthcare Cost and Utilization Project - Nationwide Inpatient Sample (HCUP-NIS), AHRQ
OA-2030-07	Reduce the rate of hospital admissions for urinary tract infections among older adults	Healthcare Cost and Utilization Project - Nationwide Inpatient Sample (HCUP-NIS), AHRQ

29. OH (Oral Health)

11 Core Objectives; 1 Developmental Objective; 0 Research Objectives

Core Objectives

Objective Number	Objective Statement	Data Source
OH-2030-01	Reduce the proportion of children and adolescents aged 3 to 19 years with lifetime tooth decay experience in their primary or permanent teeth	National Health and Nutrition Examination Survey (NHANES), CDC/NCHS
OH-2030-02	Reduce the proportion of children and adolescents aged 3 to 19 years with active and currently untreated tooth decay in their primary or permanent teeth	National Health and Nutrition Examination Survey (NHANES), CDC/NCHS
OH-2030-03	Reduce the proportion of adults aged 20 to 74 with active or currently untreated tooth decay	National Health and Nutrition Examination Survey (NHANES), CDC/NCHS
OH-2030-04	Reduce the proportion of adults aged 75 years and older with untreated root surface decay	National Health and Nutrition Examination Survey (NHANES), CDC/NCHS
OH-2030-05	Reduce the proportion of adults aged 45 and older who have lost all of their natural teeth	National Health and Nutrition Examination Survey (NHANES), CDC/NCHS
OH-2030-06	Reduce the proportion of adults aged 45 and older who have moderate and severe periodontitis	National Health and Nutrition Examination Survey (NHANES), CDC/NCHS
OH-2030-07	Increase the proportion of oral and pharyngeal cancers detected at the earliest stage	National Program of Cancer Registries (NPCR), CDC/NCCDPHP; Surveillance, Epidemiology, and End Results Program (SEER), NIH/NCI
OH-2030-08	Increase the proportion of children, adolescents, and adults who use the oral health care system	Medical Expenditure Panel Survey (MEPS), AHRQ
OH-2030-09	Increase the proportion of low income youth who have a preventive dental visit	National Survey of Children's Health (NSCH), HRSA/MCHB
OH-2030-10	Increase the proportion of children and adolescents aged 3 to 19 who have received dental sealants on one or more of their primary or permanent molar teeth	National Health and Nutrition Examination Survey (NHANES), CDC/NCHS
OH-2030-11	Increase the proportion of the U.S. population served by community systems with optimally fluoridated water systems	Water Fluoridation Reporting System (WFRS), CDC/NCCDPHP

Developmental Objectives

Objective Number	Objective Statement
OH-2030-D01	Increase the number of states and the District of Columbia that have an oral and craniofacial health surveillance system

30. Opioids

11 Core Objectives; 2 Developmental Objectives; 0 Research Objectives

Core Objectives

Objective Number	Objective Statement	Data Source
OPIOID-2030-01	Reduce overdose deaths involving natural and semisynthetic opioids (e.g., oxycodone, hydrocodone) among all persons	National Vital Statistics System-Mortality (NVSS-M), CDC/NCHS; Bridged-race Population Estimates, CDC/NCHS and Census
OPIOID-2030-02	Reduce overdose deaths involving synthetic opioids other than methadone (e.g., fentanyl) among all persons	National Vital Statistics System-Mortality (NVSS-M), CDC/NCHS; Bridged-race Population Estimates, CDC/NCHS and Census
OPIOID-2030-03	Reduce overdose deaths involving heroin among all persons	National Vital Statistics System-Mortality (NVSS-M), CDC/NCHS; Bridged-race Population Estimates, CDC/NCHS and Census
OPIOID-2030-04	Reduce the past year proportion of people ages 12 and older using heroin	National Survey on Drug Use and Health (NSDUH), SAMHSA
OPIOID-2030-05	Reduce the past year proportion of people ages 12 and older who initiate heroin use	National Survey on Drug Use and Health (NSDUH), SAMHSA
OPIOID-2030-06	Reduce the proportion of people with opioid use disorder in the past year	National Survey on Drug Use and Health (NSDUH), SAMHSA
OPIOID-2030-07	Reduce the proportion of prescription pain reliever misuse	National Survey on Drug Use and Health (NSDUH), SAMHSA
OPIOID-2030-08	Reduce the proportion of prescription pain reliever misuse initiation	National Survey on Drug Use and Health (NSDUH), SAMHSA
OPIOID-2030-09	Reduce emergency department visits for harms from nonmedical use of prescription opioids	Bridged-race Population Estimates, CDC/NCHS and Census; National Electronic Injury Surveillance System-Cooperative Adverse Drug Event Surveillance Project (NEISS-CADES), CDC and CPSC and FDA
OPIOID-2030-10	Reduce overdose deaths involving opioids among all persons	National Vital Statistics System-Mortality (NVSS-M), CDC/NCHS; Bridged-race Population Estimates, CDC/NCHS and Census

Objective Number	Objective Statement	Data Source
OPIOID-2030-11	Reduce overdose deaths involving methadone among all persons	National Vital Statistics System-Mortality (NVSS-M), CDC/NCHS; Bridged-race Population Estimates, CDC/NCHS and Census

Developmental Objectives

Objective Number	Objective Statement
OPIOID-2030-D01	Increase the rate of people with an opioid use disorder receiving medication-assisted treatment
OPIOID-2030-D02	Reduce the rate of opioid-related emergency department visits

31. OSH (Occupational Safety and Health)

7 Core Objectives; 0 Developmental Objectives; 0 Research Objectives

Core Objectives

Objective Number	Objective Statement	Data Source
OSH-2030-01	Reduce deaths from work-related injuries in all industries	Census of Fatal Occupational Injuries (CFOI), DOL/BLS; Current Population Survey (CPS), Census and DOL/BLS
OSH-2030-02	Reduce nonfatal work-related injuries resulting in one or more days away from work, as reported by employers	Survey of Occupational Injuries and Illnesses (SOII), DOL/BLS; Current Population Survey (CPS), Census and DOL/BLS
OSH-2030-03	Reduce pneumoconiosis deaths	National Vital Statistics System-Mortality (NVSS-M), CDC/NCHS
OSH-2030-04	Reduce work-related assaults	National Electronic Injury Surveillance System-Work Supplement (NEISS-WORK), CDC/NIOSH and CPSC; Current Population Survey (CPS), Census and
OSH-2030-05	Reduce the rate of elevated blood lead levels in adults with work-related lead exposure	Adult Blood Lead Epidemiology and Surveillance Program (ABLES), CDC/NIOSH
OSH-2030-06	Reduce occupational skin diseases or disorders among full-time workers	Survey of Occupational Injuries and Illnesses (SOII), DOL/BLS; Current Population Survey (CPS), Census and DOL/BLS
OSH-2030-07	Reduce new cases of occupational hearing loss	Survey of Occupational Injuries and Illnesses (SOII), DOL/BLS; Current Population Survey (CPS), Census and DOL/BLS

32. PA (Physical Activity)

11 Core Objectives; 0 Developmental Objectives; 0 Research Objectives

Core Objectives

Objective Number	Objective Statement	Data Source
PA-2030-01	Reduce the proportion of adults who engage in no leisure-time physical activity	National Health Interview Survey (NHIS), CDC/NCHS
PA-2030-02	Increase the proportion of adults who meet the current minimum aerobic physical activity guideline needed for substantial health benefits	National Health Interview Survey (NHIS), CDC/NCHS
PA-2030-03	Increase the proportion of adults who meet the current highly active aerobic physical activity guideline needed for more extensive health benefits	National Health Interview Survey (NHIS), CDC/NCHS
PA-2030-04	Increase the proportion of adults who meet the current muscle-strengthening activity guideline	National Health Interview Survey (NHIS), CDC/NCHS
PA-2030-05	Increase the proportion of adolescents who meet the current aerobic physical activity guideline	Youth Risk Behavior Surveillance System (YRBSS), CDC/NCHHSTP
PA-2030-06	Increase the proportion of adolescents who meet the current muscle-strengthening activity guideline	Youth Risk Behavior Surveillance System (YRBSS), CDC/NCHHSTP
PA-2030-07	Increase the proportion of children and adolescents aged 2 to 17 years with total screen time for no more than 2 hours a day	National Survey of Children's Health (NSCH), HRSA/MCHB
PA-2030-08	Increase the proportion of adults who walk or use a bicycle to get to and from places	National Health and Nutrition Examination Survey (NHANES), CDC/NCHS
PA-2030-09	Increase the proportion of children and adolescents aged 12 to 17 years who walk or use a bicycle to get to and from places	National Health and Nutrition Examination Survey (NHANES), CDC/NCHS
PA-2030-10	Increase the proportion of children and adolescents aged 6 to 17 years who participate on a sports team or take sports lessons after school or on weekends	National Survey of Children's Health (NSCH), HRSA/MCHB
PA-2030-11	Increase the proportion of middle and high schools that, either directly or through the school district, had a joint use agreement for shared use of school or community physical activity facilities	School Health Profiles, CDC/NCHHSTP

33. PHI (Public Health Infrastructure)

7 Core Objectives; 7 Developmental Objectives; 10 Research Objectives

Core Objectives

Objective Number	Objective Statement	Data Source
PHI-2030-01	Increase the proportion of state public health agencies that are accredited	Accredited Health Department List, Public Health Accreditation Board (PHAB)
PHI-2030-02	Increase the proportion of local public health agencies that are accredited	Accredited Health Department List, Public Health Accreditation Board (PHAB)
PHI-2030-03	Increase the number of tribal public health agencies that are accredited	Accredited Health Department List, Public Health Accreditation Board (PHAB)
PHI-2030-04	Increase the proportion of state and territorial jurisdictions that have developed a health improvement plan	ASTHO Profile of State and Territorial Public Health (ASTHO Profile), ASTHO
PHI-2030-05	Increase the proportion of local jurisdictions that have developed a health improvement plan	National Profile of Local Health Departments (NACCHO Profile), NACCHO
PHI-2030-06	Increase the proportion of state public health agencies that use Core Competencies for Public Health Professionals in continuing education for personnel	ASTHO Profile of State and Territorial Public Health (ASTHO Profile), ASTHO
PHI-2030-07	Increase the proportion of local public health agencies that use Core Competencies for Public Health Professionals in continuing education for personnel	National Profile of Local Health Departments (NACCHO Profile), NACCHO

Developmental Objectives

Objective Number	Objective Statement
PHI-2030-D01	Increase the proportion of tribal public health agencies that use Core Competencies for Public Health Professionals in continuing education for personnel
PHI-2030-D02	Increase the proportion of territorial public health agencies that use Core Competencies for Public Health Professionals in continuing education for personnel
PHI-2030-D03	Increase the proportion of vital records/health statistics programs that are nationally accredited
PHI-2030-D04	Increase the proportion of state public health laboratories that provide comprehensive laboratory services to support emerging public health issues
PHI-2030-D05	Increase the proportion of state public health laboratories that have implemented emerging technology to provide enhanced laboratory services
PHI-2030-D06	Increase the proportion of tribal communities that have developed a health improvement plan
PHI-2030-D07	Increase the proportion of territorial public health agencies that are accredited

Research Objectives

Objective Number	Objective Statement
PHI-2030-R01	Explore and expand the use and impact of practice-based continuing education resources for public health practitioners, such as training centers, learning management systems, and discipline-specific opportunities
PHI-2030-R02	Expand pipeline programs that include service learning or experiential learning components in public health settings
PHI-2030-R03	Increase use of core competencies and discipline-specific competencies to drive workforce development efforts
PHI-2030-R04	Monitor and understand the public health workforce - composition, enumeration, gaps, and needs
PHI-2030-R05	Monitor the education of the public health workforce - degrees conferred, schools and programs of public health and related disciplines, and curricula
PHI-2030-R06	Enhance informatics use and capabilities, including data-sharing and data-exchange
PHI-2030-R07	Explore the use and impact of quality improvement as a means for increasing efficiency and/or effectiveness outcomes in health departments
PHI-2030-R08	Explore financing of the public health infrastructure, including the core/foundational capabilities in health departments
PHI-2030-R09	Explore the impact of community health assessment and improvement planning efforts on resource allocation, partnerships, community needs, and health outcomes

Objective Number	Objective Statement
PHI-2030-R10	Explore the impact of accreditation and national standards on health department performance and community health outcomes

34. PREP (Preparedness)

2 Core Objectives; 4 Developmental Objectives; 0 Research Objectives

Core Objectives

Objective Number	Objective Statement	Data Source
PREP-2030-01	Increase the rate of bystander CPR for all non-traumatic cardiac arrests	Cardiac Arrest Registry to Enhance Survival (CARES), Emory University
PREP-2030-02	Increase the rate of bystander automated external defibrillator (AED) use for non-traumatic cardiac arrests occurring in public locations	Cardiac Arrest Registry to Enhance Survival (CARES), Emory University

Developmental Objectives

Objective Number	Objective Statement
PREP-2030-D01	Increase the proportion of parents and/or guardians aware of the emergency or evacuation plan in their child(ren)'s school including the evacuation location and how to get information about the child in the event of a disaster
PREP-2030-D02	Increase the proportion of adults who engage in preparedness activities for a widespread outbreak of a contagious disease after recently receiving preparedness information on outbreaks
PREP-2030-D03	Increase the proportion of adults who are aware of their transportation support needs to evacuate in preparation of a hurricane, flood, or wildfire
PREP-2030-D04	Increase the proportion of adults whose household has an emergency plan that includes instructions for household members, including at-risk individuals, about where to go and what to do in the event of a disaster

35. RD (Respiratory Diseases)

6 Core Objectives; 4 Developmental Objectives; 0 Research Objectives

Core Objectives

Objective Number	Objective Statement	Data Source
RD-2030-01	Reduce asthma deaths among the U.S. population	National Vital Statistics System-Mortality (NVSS-M), CDC/NCHS; Bridged-race Population Estimates, CDC/NCHS and Census
RD-2030-02	Reduce emergency department visits for children with asthma under 5 years	National Hospital Ambulatory Medical Care Survey (NHAMCS), CDC/NCHS; Population Estimates,
RD-2030-03	Reduce emergency department visits for persons with asthma aged ≥ 5 years	National Hospital Ambulatory Medical Care Survey (NHAMCS), CDC/NCHS; Population Estimates,
RD-2030-04	Reduce deaths from chronic obstructive pulmonary disease (COPD) among adults	National Vital Statistics System-Mortality (NVSS-M), CDC/NCHS; Bridged-race Population Estimates, CDC/NCHS and Census
RD-2030-05	Reduce emergency department visits for chronic obstructive pulmonary disease (COPD)	National Hospital Ambulatory Medical Care Survey (NHAMCS), CDC/NCHS; Population Estimates,
RD-2030-06	Reduce asthma attacks among persons with current asthma	National Health Interview Survey (NHIS), CDC/NCHS

Developmental Objectives

Objective Number	Objective Statement
RD-2030-D01	Reduce hospitalizations for asthma among children under age 5 years
RD-2030-D02	Reduce hospitalizations for asthma among children and adults aged 5 to 64 years
RD-2030-D03	Reduce hospitalizations for asthma among adults aged 65 years and older
RD-2030-D04	Reduce hospitalizations for chronic obstructive pulmonary disease (COPD)

36. SDOH (Social Determinants of Health)

6 Core Objectives; 0 Developmental Objectives; 1 Research Objective

Core Objectives

Objective Number	Objective Statement	Data Source
SDOH-2030-01	Increase the proportion of children aged 0-17 years living with at least one parent employed year round, full time	Current Population Survey (CPS), Census and DOL/BLS
SDOH-2030-02	Increase the proportion of high school completers who were enrolled in college the October immediately after completing high school	Current Population Survey (CPS), Census and DOL/BLS
SDOH-2030-03	Reduce the proportion of persons living in poverty	Current Population Survey (CPS), Census and
SDOH-2030-04	Reduce the proportion of all households that spend more than 30 percent of income on housing	American Housing Survey, HUD and Census
SDOH-2030-05	Reduce the proportion of children who had ever experienced a parent who has served time in jail	National Survey of Children's Health (NSCH), HRSA/MCHB
SDOH-2030-06	Increase employment among working-age individuals, ages 16-64	Current Population Survey (CPS), Census and

Research Objectives

Objective Number	Objective Statement
SDOH-2030-R01	Increase the proportion of federal data sources that collect country of birth as a variable

37. SH (Sleep Health)

4 Core Objectives; 0 Developmental Objectives; 0 Research Objectives

Core Objectives

Objective	Objective Statement	Data Source
SH-2030-01	Reduce the rate of vehicular crashes that are due to drowsy driving	Crash Report Sampling System (CRSS), DOT/NHTSA
SH-2030-02	Increase the proportion of persons with symptoms of obstructive sleep apnea who seek medical evaluation	National Health and Nutrition Examination Survey (NHANES), CDC/NCHS
SH-2030-03	Increase the proportion of adults who get sufficient sleep	National Health Interview Survey (NHIS), CDC/NCHS
SH-2030-04	Increase the proportion of students in grades 9 through 12 who get sufficient sleep	Youth Risk Behavior Surveillance System (YRBSS), CDC/NCHHSTP

38. STD (Sexually Transmitted Diseases)

6 Core Objectives; 1 Developmental Objective; 0 Research Objectives

Core Objectives

Objective Number	Objective Statement	Data Source
STD-2030-01	Increase the proportion of sexually active females aged 16 to 24 years enrolled in Medicaid and commercial health plans who are screened for chlamydial infections	Healthcare Effectiveness Data and Information Set (HEDIS), NCQA
STD-2030-02	Reduce gonorrhea rates among males aged 15 to 24 years	National Notifiable Diseases Surveillance System (NNDSS), CDC/PHSIPO
STD-2030-03	Reduce the incidence of primary and secondary syphilis in women aged 15-44	National Notifiable Diseases Surveillance System (NNDSS), CDC/PHSIPO
STD-2030-04	Reduce congenital syphilis	National Notifiable Diseases Surveillance System (NNDSS), CDC/PHSIPO
STD-2030-05	Reduce pelvic inflammatory disease in women aged 15-24 years	National Disease and Therapeutic Index (NDTI)
STD-2030-06	Reduce the proportion of population aged 15-24 with herpes simplex virus-2	National Health and Nutrition Examination Survey (NHANES), CDC/NCHS

Developmental Objectives

Objective Number	Objective Statement
STD-2030-D01	Reduce the rate of primary and secondary syphilis in men who have sex with men

39. SU (Substance Use)

15 Core Objectives; 2 Developmental Objectives; 1 Research Objective

Core Objectives

Objective Number	Objective Statement	Data Source
SU-2030-01	Increase the proportion of persons who need alcohol and/or illicit drug treatment and received specialty treatment for substance use problem in the past year	National Survey on Drug Use and Health (NSDUH), SAMHSA
SU-2030-02	Reduce cirrhosis deaths	Bridged-race Population Estimates, CDC/NCHS and Census; National Vital Statistics System-Mortality (NVSS-M), CDC/NCHS
SU-2030-03	Reduce drug overdose deaths	Bridged-race Population Estimates, CDC/NCHS and Census; National Vital Statistics System-Mortality (NVSS-M), CDC/NCHS
SU-2030-04	Reduce the proportion of adolescents reporting use of alcohol during the past 30 days	National Survey on Drug Use and Health (NSDUH), SAMHSA
SU-2030-05	Reduce the proportion of adolescents reporting use of any illicit drugs during the past 30 days	National Survey on Drug Use and Health (NSDUH), SAMHSA
SU-2030-06	Reduce the proportion of adolescents reporting use of marijuana in the past 30 days	National Survey on Drug Use and Health (NSDUH), SAMHSA
SU-2030-07	Reduce the proportion of adults reporting use of any illicit drug during the past 30 days	National Survey on Drug Use and Health (NSDUH), SAMHSA
SU-2030-08	Reduce the proportion of adults reporting use of marijuana daily or almost daily	National Survey on Drug Use and Health (NSDUH), SAMHSA
SU-2030-09	Reduce the proportion of persons under 21 engaging in binge drinking of alcoholic beverages	National Survey on Drug Use and Health (NSDUH), SAMHSA
SU-2030-10	Reduce the proportion of persons 21 and older engaging in binge drinking of alcoholic beverages	National Survey on Drug Use and Health (NSDUH), SAMHSA
SU-2030-11	Reduce the proportion of motor vehicle crash deaths involving an alcohol-impaired driver with a blood alcohol concentration (BAC) of 0.08 g/dL or higher	Fatality Analysis Reporting System (FARS), DOT/NHTSA

Objective Number	Objective Statement	Data Source
SU-2030-12	Reduce the past-year misuse of prescription drugs	National Survey on Drug Use and Health (NSDUH), SAMHSA
SU-2030-13	Reduce the proportion of people with alcohol use disorder in the past year	National Survey on Drug Use and Health (NSDUH), SAMHSA
SU-2030-14	Reduce the proportion of people with marijuana use disorder in the past year	National Survey on Drug Use and Health (NSDUH), SAMHSA
SU-2030-15	Reduce the proportion of people with an illicit drug use disorder in the past year	National Survey on Drug Use and Health (NSDUH), SAMHSA

Developmental Objectives

Objective Number	Objective Statement
SU-2030-D01	Increase the number of admissions to substance abuse treatment for injection drug use
SU-2030-D02	Increase the proportion of persons who are referred for follow up care for alcohol problems, drug problems after diagnosis, or treatment for one of these conditions in a hospital emergency department

Research Objectives

Objective Number	Objective Statement
SU-2030-R01	Increase the proportion of adolescents who perceive great risk associated with substance abuse

40. TU (Tobacco Use)

20 Core Objectives; 0 Developmental Objectives; 0 Research Objectives

Core Objectives

Objective Number	Objective Statement	Data Source
TU-2030-01	Reduce current use of any tobacco products among adults	National Health Interview Survey (NHIS), CDC/NCHS
TU-2030-02	Reduce current use of cigarettes among adults	National Health Interview Survey (NHIS), CDC/NCHS
TU-2030-03	Reduce current use of any tobacco products among adolescents	National Youth Tobacco Survey (NYTS), CDC/NCCDPHP
TU-2030-04	Reduce current use of e-cigarettes among adolescents	National Youth Tobacco Survey (NYTS), CDC/NCCDPHP
TU-2030-05	Reduce current use of cigarettes among adolescents	National Youth Tobacco Survey (NYTS), CDC/NCCDPHP
TU-2030-06	Reduce current use of cigars, cigarillos and little cigars among adolescents	National Youth Tobacco Survey (NYTS), CDC/NCCDPHP
TU-2030-07	Reduce current use of flavored tobacco products among adolescent tobacco users	National Youth Tobacco Survey (NYTS), CDC/NCCDPHP
TU-2030-08	Reduce the initiation of the use of cigarettes among adolescents and young adults	National Survey on Drug Use and Health (NSDUH), SAMHSA
TU-2030-09	Increase smoking quit attempts among adult smokers (past year)	National Health Interview Survey (NHIS), CDC/NCHS
TU-2030-10	Increase the proportion of adult smokers who receive advice to quit from a health professional	National Health Interview Survey (NHIS) Cancer Control Supplement, CDC/NCHS
TU-2030-11	Increase use of smoking cessation counseling and/or medication among adult smokers	National Health Interview Survey (NHIS) Cancer Control Supplement, CDC/NCHS
TU-2030-12	Increase recent smoking cessation success among adult smokers	National Health Interview Survey (NHIS), CDC/NCHS
TU-2030-13	Increase smoking cessation during pregnancy among females	National Vital Statistics System (NVSS), CDC/NCHS
TU-2030-14	Increase the number of states, the District of Columbia, and territories that have smoke-free policies that prohibit smoking in all indoor areas of worksites, restaurants and bars	State Tobacco Activities Tracking and Evaluation System (STATE), CDC/NCCDPHP

Objective Number	Objective Statement	Data Source
TU-2030-15	Increase the number of states, the District of Columbia, and territories that have smoke-free policies that prohibit smoking in all indoor areas of multiunit housing	State Tobacco Activities Tracking and Evaluation System (STATE), CDC/NCCDPHP
TU-2030-16	Increase the proportion of smoke free homes	Tobacco Use Supplement-Current Population Survey (TUS-CPS); Census, DOL/BLS, NIH/NCI, FDA/CTP
TU-2030-17	Reduce the proportion of children, adolescents and adults exposed to secondhand smoke	National Health and Nutrition Examination Survey (NHANES), CDC/NCHS
TU-2030-18	Increase the national average tax on cigarettes	State Tobacco Activities Tracking and Evaluation System (STATE), CDC/NCCDPHP
TU-2030-19	Reduce the proportion of adolescents in grades 6-12 who are exposed to tobacco product marketing	National Youth Tobacco Survey (NYTS), CDC/NCCDPHP
TU-2030-20	Increase the number of states, the District of Columbia, and territories that establish 21 years as the minimum age for purchasing tobacco products	State Tobacco Activities Tracking and Evaluation System (STATE), CDC/NCCDPHP

41. V (Vision)

9 Core Objectives; 1 Developmental Objective; 0 Research

Objectives Core Objectives

Objective Number	Objective Statement	Data Source
V-2030-01	Increase the proportion of preschool children aged 3-5 years who receive vision screening	National Health Interview Survey (NHIS), CDC/NCHS
V-2030-02	Increase the proportion of adults who have a comprehensive eye examination, including dilation, within the past 2 years	National Health Interview Survey (NHIS), CDC/NCHS
V-2030-03	Reduce blindness and visual impairment in children and adolescents aged 17 years and under	National Health Interview Survey (NHIS), CDC/NCHS
V-2030-04	Reduce visual impairment due to diabetic retinopathy	National Health Interview Survey (NHIS), CDC/NCHS
V-2030-05	Reduce visual impairment due to glaucoma	National Health Interview Survey (NHIS), CDC/NCHS
V-2030-06	Reduce visual impairment due to cataract	National Health Interview Survey (NHIS), CDC/NCHS
V-2030-07	Reduce visual impairment due to age-related macular degeneration	National Health Interview Survey (NHIS), CDC/NCHS
V-2030-08	Increase the use of vision rehabilitation services by persons with visual impairment	National Health Interview Survey (NHIS), CDC/NCHS
V-2030-09	Increase the use of assistive and adaptive devices by persons with visual impairment	National Health Interview Survey (NHIS), CDC/NCHS

Developmental Objectives

Objective Number	Objective Statement
V-2030-D01	Reduce visual impairment due to uncorrected refractive error